Get Through

MRCOG Part 1

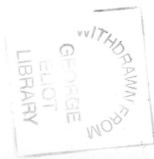

To Christine, Laura, Alice, Joseph and Eleanor (TJC)

To Dukaydah, Abdea and Tara (AC)

Get Through
MRCOG Part 2: OSCE

T. Justin Clark MD (Hons) MRCOG
Consultant Obstetrician and Gynaecologist and Honorary Senior Lecturer,
Birmingham Women's Hospital and University of Birmingham, Birmingham

Arri Coomarasamy MD MRCOG
Subspecialist Trainee in Reproductive Medicine and Surgery,
Senior Registrar in Obstetrics and Gynaecology and
Honorary Lecturer in Clinical Epidemiology,
Guy's and St Thomas' NHS Trust, London

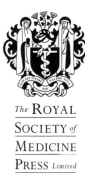

The ROYAL
SOCIETY *of*
MEDICINE
PRESS Limited

© 2008 Royal Society of Medicine Ltd
Published by the Royal Society of Medicine Press Ltd
1 Wimpole Street, London W1G 0AE, UK
Tel: +44 (0)20 7290 2921
Fax: +44 (0)20 7290 2929
E-mail: publishing@rsmpress.co.uk

British Library Cataloguing in Publication Data
A catalogue record for this book is available from the British Library

ISBN: 978-1-85315-721-9

Distribution in Europe and Rest of the World:
Marston Book Services Ltd
PO Box 269
Abingdon
Oxon OX14 4YN, UK
Tel: +44 (0)1235 465500
Fax: +44 (0)1235 465555
Email: direct.order@marston.co.uk

Distribution in USA and Canada:
Royal Society of Medicine Press Ltd
c/o BookMasters Inc
30 Amberwood Parkway
Ashland, OH 44805, USA
Tel: +1 800 247 6553/ +1 800 266 5564
Fax: +1 410 281 6883
Email: order@bookmasters.com

Distribution in Australia and New Zealand:
Elsevier Australia
30–52 Smidmore Street
Marrickville NSW 2204, Australia
Tel: +61 2 9517 8999
Fax: +61 2 9517 2249
Email: service@elsevier.com.au

Typeset by Phoenix Photosetting, Chatham, Kent
Printed in the UK by Bell & Bain Ltd, Glasgow

Contents

About the authors

T. Justin Clark MD (Hons) MRCOG is a Consultant Obstetrician and Gynaecologist at the Birmingham Women's Hospital. He also has close links with Birmingham University where he is an Honorary Senior Lecturer and Clinical Subdean. He is involved both with designing and delivering undergraduate and postgraduate training programmes and teaches on MBChB and MRCOG courses utilizing his expertise in evidence-based medicine. His clinical and research interests lie in minimal access surgery where he holds over £1 million in research funding. He lectures internationally and has published widely in this area.

Arri Coomarasamy MD MRCOG is a Subspecialist Trainee in Reproductive Medicine and Surgery, and a Senior Registrar in Obstetrics and Gynaecology at Guy's and St Thomas' Hospitals. He holds numerous research grants, of over £3 million, and has published over 70 peer-reviewed articles. He has extensive experience in organizing and delivering courses for MRCOG, DRCOG and evidence-based medicine. He is an editor for BJOG, and a trustee of Ammalife, an international charity with a mission to reduce maternal death and disability in the developing world (www.ammalife.org).

Foreword

The MRCOG examination is a core part of the training to be an Obstetrician and Gynaecologist. It is a knowledge-based examination and, together with training within a clinical programme, forms a crucial part in preparing young doctors for the rigour of senior posts in Obstetrics and Gynaecology, both in the UK and overseas. Passing the examination is necessary to progress in the training programme within the UK; indeed, without the MRCOG trainees cannot progress to the last 2 years of senior training, where they learn the important special skills that will equip them to work as senior doctors.

The Part 2 examination comprises a multiple choice and extended matching question paper, together with two short answer papers; having passed this part candidates go onto sit the OSCE component of the examination. While OSCEs are increasingly familiar to our trainees, there remains a fear and anxiety about this type of examination. Trainees are often ill at ease when in a station with an actor and an impassive examiner, and find the situation strange and difficult. These stations are very necessary to test the all important communications skills of candidates and their ability to apply their knowledge in an often very difficult and stressful clinical situation.

Preparation is crucial and there are very many ways to prepare for the OSCE. Courses are important but are limited by availability and time. This book, with its clear layout and simple pragmatic approach, is an excellent resource for candidates; providing a useful number of examples of stations combined with sensible and practical advice about how to approach them. Reading this book will enable candidates to understand the principles underpinning the OSCE and be better prepared to sit the examination.

Dr Maggie Blott
Consultant Obstetrician, University College London Hospitals;
Vice President for Education,
Royal College of Obstetricians and Gynaecologists

Preface

We have written this book primarily as a response to requests from delegates who have attended our long-established and successful 'ACE' MRCOG II OSCE course (www.acecourses.co.uk). The book is based upon our experience of designing and delivering this course, and the feedback we have received from the past candidates over the years. We appreciate candidates often have hundreds of questions that they have gathered from past exams and there is a multitude of OSCE books out there already. Our intention is not to provide another book that mindlessly catalogues dozens and dozens of questions. Our aims are deeper – we wish to give you *insights* on what makes some candidates stand out, and we want to provide you with the techniques, tools and frameworks that will allow you to tackle most questions with ease. In short, we do not simply want to give you some fish, but teach you how to fish for yourself.

It is all very well when well-meaning colleagues or tutors tell you that you must 'empathize' when dealing with an angry patient, but what exactly does that mean? They tell you to use a 'structured approach' when you appraise an article or an audit, or even when you take a history, but what are these structures? They tell you your revision needs to be 'focused', but just how do you get focused? They tell you that you must have a 'strategy' when things are not going according to plan in the exam, but what is this strategy? They tell you 'communication skills' are what win the day, but can these be learned? Our book gives you practical guidance on these and many other burning questions on techniques.

In our OSCE courses, candidates have often invited us to answer questions such as: How do I explain a 'molar pregnancy' or 'gastroschisis' to the patient (role player)? Should I greet the examiner? How do I deal with a difficult consultation? How can I compose myself if I perform badly on a station? How do I describe surgical instruments, procedures or results of investigation? What is the best way to approach a clinical prioritization station? You will find the answers to these and other questions in this book.

We hope you find the material presented useful and a key part of your preparation and ultimate success in achieving membership of the Royal College of Obstetricians and Gynaecologists. We welcome your feedback, please contact us at publishing@rsm.ac.uk.

T. Justin Clark
Arri Coomarasamy

Acknowledgement

We thank Dr Pallavi Latthe for writing the OSCE question on urodynamic investigation.

Abbreviations

5-FU	5-fluorouracil
ABG	arterial blood gas
AFB	aflatoxin B
AFLP	acute fatty liver of pregnancy
APH	antepartum haemorrhage
ARM	assisted rupture of membranes
ART	artificial reproductive technique
BMI	body mass index
BNA	borderline nuclear abnormality
BSO	bilateral salpingo-oophorectomy
CBT	cognitive behavioural therapy
CI	confidence interval
COC	combined oral contraceptive
CRL	crown–rump length
C/S	caesarean section
CT	computerised tomography
CTG	cardiotograph
CVA	cerebrovascular accident
CVP	central venous pressure
CXR	chest X-ray
DMPA	Depo medroxyprogesterone acetate
DOA	detrusor overactivity
DUB	dysfunctional uterine bleeding
EAS	external anal sphincter
EBL	estimated blood loss
ECV	external cephalic version
EFM	electronic fetal monitoring
EFW	estimated fetal weight
ERPC	evacuation of retained products of conception
ERT	(o)estrogen replacement therapy
FBC	full blood count
FBS	fetal blood sample
FFP	fresh frozen plasma
FHR	fetal heart rate
FSH	follicle stimulating hormone
GA	general anaesthesia
GIT	gastrointestinal

G&S group and save
GTT glucose tolerance test
GU genitourinary
hCG human chorionic gonadotrophin
HDU high dependency unit
HPV human papilloma virus
HRQL health-related quality of life
HRT hormone replacement therapy
HVS high vaginal swab
IAS internal anal sphincter
ICSI intracytoplasmic sperm injection
ICU intensive care unit
IHD ischaemic heart disease
IMB intermenstrual bleeding
IOL induction of labour
IPV internal podalic version
IUCD intrauterine contraceptive device
IUGR intrauterine growth retardation
IUI intrauterine insemination
IVU intravenous urogram
LAVH laparoscopic assisted vaginal hysterectomy
LH luteinizing hormone
LFT liver function test
LGT lower genital tract
LMP last menstrual period
LMWH low molecular weight heparin
LOA left occiputo-anterior
LOP left occiputo-posterior
LUS lower uterine segment
LW labour ward
MDT multidisciplinary team
MRI magnetic resonance imaging
MRSA methicillin-resistant *Staphylococcus aureus*
MSU midstream urine
NAD no abnormality detected
NBM nil by mouth
NNT number needed to treat
NTD neural tube defect
NVD normal vaginal delivery
OA occipito-anterior
OCP oral contraceptive pill

OP	occipito-posterior
OT	occipito-transverse
PBC	primary biliary cirrhosis
PCB	postcoital bleeding
PCO	polycystic ovaries
PE	pulmonary embolism
PET	positron emission tomography
PID	pelvic inflammatory disease
PMB	post-menopausal bleeding
PMH	past medical history
PMS	premenstrual syndrome
POP	progestogen-only pill
PPH	postpartum haemorrhage
PTL	preterm labour
RCT	randomized controlled trial
RPOC	retained products of conception
RR	relative risk
RTI	reproductive tract infection
RV	rectovaginal
SFA	seminal fluid analysis
SFH	symphysial fundal height
SOB	shortness of breath
SPD	symphysis pubis dysfunction
SROM	spontaneous rupture of membranes
STI	sexually transmitted infection
TAH	total abdominal hysterectomy
TOP	termination of pregnancy
TVS	transvaginal scan
TVT	transvaginal tape
U&E	urea and electrolytes
UDCA	ursodeoxycholic acid
USS	ultrasound scan
VE	venous embolism
VI	virgo intacta
VIN	vulval intraepithelial neoplasia
VTE	venous thromboembolism
VVF	vesico-vaginal fistula
WLE	wide local incision

Introduction

You have passed your MRCOG Part 1 and Part 2 written exams. These exams have surely examined you in depth. Why an OSCE? The reason is that your written exams predominantly assess your knowledge, and to a lesser extent the application of *knowledge* (especially with the advent of EMQs), but do not offer an assessment of your *skills, attitudes* and *behaviour.* An OSCE exam would allow the examination of some of these higher dimensions. It is often clichéd, but is probably true, that the examiners in an OSCE exam are primarily seeking to answer the questions: 'Would I want this doctor as my registrar?' or 'Would I like to be cared for by a doctor like this?' Thus the focus is no longer on exhibiting your prowess in knowledge, but your holistic, sensitive, caring and safe approach to the care of your patients.

OSCEs are objective and structured, which is to say that everyone gets the same questions, and marking is according to a pre-set marking scheme. According to the current format, you will get 12 questions (with two preparatory stations), thus offering a wide sampling across the topic areas in O&G. You have 15 minutes per question, which is generally split into 14 minutes for answering and 1 minute for marking. Thus the total duration of the exam is 3 hours. The marking is criterion-referenced (and not norm-referenced), i.e. the pass mark (minimum standard) is pre-set and does not depend on how well the other candidates do.

This book has been written to help you succeed in passing the MRCOG Part 2 OSCE. We have concentrated upon the techniques that are required to handle specific OSCE stations, key information that is not generally available from traditional textbooks. We hope that the book acts as a sound basis for your exam preparation, providing familiarity with the exam and focusing revision and practice on relevant areas. As described above the examiners in an OSCE

1

exam are primarily seeking to answer simple questions about your competence. Thus, if the exam is to be valid it should be passed by all bright, hardworking and caring young doctors. If you are such a doctor, then, with adequate preparation, you will ultimately overcome this professional hurdle and pass. May we wish you the best of luck.

Section 1

Preparation for the MRCOG Part 2 OSCE

1 Preparation for the MRCOG Part 2 OSCE

There is certainly a right and a wrong way to prepare for the OSCE. Some potential elements of the 'right way' are detailed below. The most important element of the 'wrong way' is an undue focus on building your knowledge base by reading thick volumes of textbooks. Remind yourself: this exam is not primarily about knowledge, but about attitudes, skills and behaviour. Your didactic textbooks are unlikely to help.

Practical preparation

Know your exam

Ensure familiarity with the exam by making sure that you are clear regarding the OSCE format. Talking to candidates who have sat the exam recently, asking the advice of a senior colleague, re-reading the course syllabus, reviewing past papers and reading an OSCE revision book or attending Part 2 OSCE courses will generally help focus your energy in the right place and help psyche yourself up. Read the MRCOG Examination Regulations on www.rcog.org.uk if you have not read them already.

Know your syllabus

Again, consult the RCOG website.

Develop and stick to a strategy

This means regular practice and setting an achievable schedule. You should aim to do short but regular studying/practice sessions rather than trying to process large quantities of information rapidly, i.e. 'cramming'. The OSCE is a practical test and so 'practice' rather than 'book work' is what is required. Most of our candidates tell us that they spend about 3 hours a day preparing for the OSCE. You may decide that you will spend ½ an hour every day reading and 1 hour practising OSCEs by yourself, and another hour for 'group practice'. It does not generally matter what your exact strategy is, but you must have a strategy and its predominant component should be practising OSCE questions.

Study groups or partners

Preparing for an exam can be a lonely experience. Identifying a study partner or partners can be valuable to many candidates because they can pick up tips from peers, and learn from other's good (or bad!) performance. In addition, study groups can increase the efficiency of learning, especially as you can share tasks such as arranging clinical teaching sessions. Interaction with colleagues in a similar position can make study more enjoyable and help maintain motivation.

When you have a 'group practice' session, set an agenda before starting, e.g. if there are three of you, you can decide that over 1½ hours you will do two questions each, thus covering a total of six stations. Be sure you choose your revision partners carefully, and emulate exam conditions as far as possible (with a stopwatch to keep an eye on the time, and marking using a structured pre-set marking scheme). Our recommendation is that there should not generally be more than three in a study group (to ensure each of you gets sufficient individual exposure to questions).

Choose your learning materials carefully

Identify, assemble and locate all relevant source materials (OSCE revision books, course materials, notes), which will avoid frustration, panic and wasting time trying to find revision material. At this stage, it is important *not* to spend your time with books that aim to impart knowledge, often to a deeper level than you require for the OSCE. In our opinion, these include the many heavy textbooks, RCOG Year books, Progress series and Advances series. Instead, our recommendations are:

- Patient information leaflets (from your hospital, RCOG website, NHS Direct website);
- RCOG guidelines and executive summaries of relevant NICE and SIGN guidelines;
- MRCOG OSCE revision books;
- *BJOG* and *BMJ* reviews and commentaries (but not primary articles).

Arrange meetings

You should arrange meetings with the following people:

- Paediatrician/neonatologist: Ask them to take you through the routine examination of the newborn. Have a list of topics to quiz them on, e.g. how do you deal with a jaundiced baby? Ask them to take you through neonatal resuscitation.
- Theatre nurse. Ask them to take you through theatre instruments. Assemble and disassemble the instruments.
- Bereavement nurse. Ask if you can sit in during consultations. Do a role play with them.
- Your local STI specialist.
- Your local family planning clinic.

Mental and physical preparation for the examination

We are all used to spending hours studying or 'cramming' prior to any examination. However, whilst acquiring knowledge is an important component of exam preparation, it is not the only one. Optimal performance requires attention to psychological and physical preparation.

Motivation

Create a schedule and stick to it. As with resolutions to diet, exercise or quit smoking, it is easier to maintain interest in these 'programmes' once a positive start has been made and the results start to show. Make a conscious decision to start early.

Allow time for leisure and relaxation

The majority of you will be busy practising clinicians with on-call commitments and some of you may have families to look after. The anxiety and time involved with exam preparation can become overwhelming if you are not careful. Setting aside personal time is crucial to your welfare and mental preparation. Spending time relaxing, exercising and with family or friends will reduce anxiety and put the importance of the exam in perspective.

Exercise and diet

Exercising regularly can help clear your mind, reduce stress and increase the effectiveness of your revision by improving mental alertness and concentration, reducing fatigue and ensuring a better night's sleep. Studying will improve if you can maintain a balanced diet and avoid heavy meals that are likely to make you feel sluggish and bloated.

Relaxation techniques

The authors do not have great familiarity with relaxation techniques, but many friends and colleagues swear by them. Techniques involve finding a quiet place and taking 20 minutes or so to practise deep breathing techniques and muscle exercises (tensing and relaxing different muscle groups), visualization and centring activities, meditation, success imagery and progressive relaxation techniques. If investing time in these activities is not for you, then listening to music, soaking in the bath or an invigorating walk are just as good.

Strategic and mental planning

This book will provide you with valuable information regarding techniques and approaches to individual OSCE stations and the overall OSCE circuit. There are often different ways to approach a station, e.g. the order of history taking, presentation of labour ward prioritization, and so on. The crucial issue is that you do not just 'decide on the day' the strategy that you will employ. Plan your approach in advance. Some authorities describe the use of 'guided imagery' or 'creative visualization' as a means of preparation, which involves visualizing the exam venue and circuit, starting the exam, how you will approach each station, etc.

Strategies if things 'go wrong'

With good preparation the chances of things going wrong or feeling overwhelmed by the test are minimized and you will pass the MRCOG Part 2. However, even the most able, well-prepared candidate can have a bad question, a bad station or a moment of mental 'blankness'. Do not panic! Plan how you are going to deal with such a situation should it arise. Different approaches work for different people, e.g. pausing and asking the examiner for a few seconds to collect your thoughts, closing your eyes and breathing deeply, asking for questions to be rephrased or time to re-read the instructions. Remember, some stations may not go as planned and you can still pass. The key is to put any station that does not go well out of you mind immediately and to approach the next station with a positive attitude. Prepare yourself up for this eventuality beforehand.

The night before

You mother was right! The best thing to do is to stop working, relax and get a good night's sleep. Make sure you have a light breakfast and dress smartly to instill self-confidence.

Practical arrangements

Be clear of the times and location of the exam, orientate yourself, plan transport and accommodation, and allow plenty of time to arrive on time. Do not talk about specifics of the exam beforehand as anxiety can be contagious!

Section 2

Techniques for specific OSCE stations

2 History and management stations

The 'history and management' stations are a good opportunity for the clinically experienced candidate to shine. The majority of MRCOG Part 2 candidates will already have a few years of valuable clinical experience under their belts such that taking a relevant patient history, conducting an appropriate examination, arriving at a diagnosis and formulating a management plan are second nature. The ability to interact with the patient and to elicit important information represents some of the 'art' of medicine, whereas assimilating, interpreting and applying this received information represents more of the 'science' of medicine. As busy clinicians you undertake this clinical process (Figure 2.1) implicitly in an often seamless fashion. In the context of the postgraduate clinical examination however, you need to display explicitly these fundamental clinical abilities to a third party. This requirement can sometimes throw the otherwise clinically competent candidate. Thus, as with all facets of the MRCOG Part 2 OSCE, an understanding of the station's requirements will allow suitable approaches to be developed and practised. Optimal performance requires preparation, even by the most clinically competent of candidates.

FIGURE 2.1   The clinical process

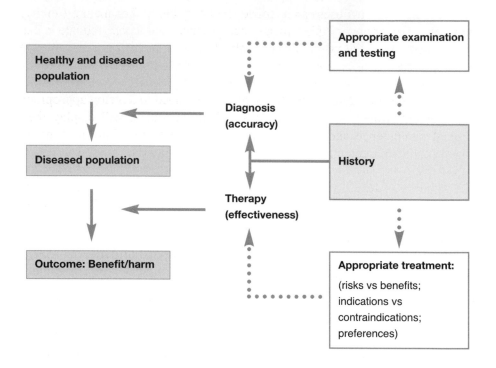

Taking a patient history

You all learnt the process of history taking as medical students and most of you will have had this generic skill observed and examined during your undergraduate years. As postgraduates, you are taught new practical skills and your competency is assessed. The ability to take a history, however, is invariably 'taken as read' and consequently this most fundamental and crucial clinical skill is overlooked. From running clinical courses and examining MRCOG Part 2 candidates, it is surprising how many candidates perform poorly when asked to take and present a succinct clinical history. Nothing raises an examiner's 'antibodies' more than being forced to sit through a prolonged, largely irrelevant and convoluted history! (You can experience the feeling for yourself by asking a representative group of medical students to take and present histories to you.) In contrast, a confident, well taken, relevant and clearly presented history is a pleasure to witness and in practice the examiner may 'switch off' after the first minute as a result of the great first impression.

The main purpose of history taking is to aid the clinician in establishing a diagnosis (or certainly a list of diagnostic possibilities). It has been estimated that over 70% of diagnoses can be made on history alone. The main difference between a patient history taken by an undergraduate and a postgraduate is that the history has a 'purpose', i.e. it is the first and most important step in acquiring the clinical diagnosis so that appropriate treatments can be instituted. Medical students often consider treating a condition in an abstract way with little consideration for the patient or the need to develop appropriate management strategies. The good postgraduate candidate will display their clinical competence and maturity by taking these factors into account. In addition, a good interaction with the patient whilst obtaining a clinical history allows the doctor to develop a rapport with their patient, relate the history to the patient's health-related quality of life (HRQL) and direct the relevant physical examination, subsequent investigations and treatment. Try to convey empathy and confidence, thereby engendering a feeling of trust in your patients (and your examiner!) in your abilities.

In order to ensure a good performance, the following points should be considered and more importantly practised:

- **Preparation** – read the question carefully and consider what the station is testing and what the likely diagnoses may be. Before entering the station, think about your introduction and opening few questions (a confident, enthusiastic, clear start ensures a good first impression and allows nerves to dissipate, improving subsequent performance).
- **Introduction** – confident, clear and engage the patient (pleasant manner, eye contact, etc).
- **Structure of history** – There are different approaches to obtaining a patient history. The aim is to obtain an efficient, comprehensive and relevant history in a logical sequence. The order of taking the history does not really matter as long as this aim is achieved. Standard structures for O&G histories are shown below.

Standard structures for history taking in O&G

Obstetric history

- Presenting complaint
- History of presenting complaint
- History of current pregnancy
- Past obstetric history
- Past medical history
- Drug history
- Family history
- Social history

Obstetric history summary (template)

Mrs NAME is a AGE-year-old OCCUPATION presenting at NUMBER OF WEEKS' gestation in her NUMBER pregnancy with PRESENTING COMPLAINT (DURATION). Additional sentence(s) – add any relevant risk factors, investigation results, diagnoses and management to date

Gynaecological history

- Presenting complaint
- History of presenting complaint
- Systematic enquiry
- Past obstetric history
- Past medical history
- Drug history
- Family history
- Social history

Gynaecological history summary (template)

Mrs NAME is a AGE-year-old OCCUPATION presenting with PRESENTING COMPLAINT (DURATION). Additional sentence(s) – add any relevant risk factors, investigation results, diagnoses and management to date

---

Important points in the obstetric history

- **Context** – LMP (estimated date of delivery); gravidity + parity.
- **Presenting complaint (duration).**
- **History of presenting complaint:**
  - Include onset, duration, progress, management, relevant symptoms and related risk factors for particular symptoms (this demonstrates to the examiner your understanding of potential diagnoses; important 'negative' answers are as important as positive responses);
  - Fetal movements.
- **History of current pregnancy:**
  - *Pre-pregnancy* (e.g. folic acid, rubella status, diabetic control); diagnosis of pregnancy; early pregnancy problems (bleeding, vomiting); gestation at booking; routine investigations (booking bloods, screening tests and scans);
  - *Antenatal care to date* (including plans of care, e.g. additional scans, day assessment unit appointments, glucose tolerance tests and emergency attendances/admissions).

- **Past obstetric history:**
  - *Chronological* – year of delivery and duration of pregnancy;
  - *Gravidity* – miscarriage/termination/ectopic – diagnosis and management;
  - *Parity* – onset of labour (induced or spontaneous); mode of delivery, reason for operative delivery, birth weight; gender; complications (antenatal, perinatal or postnatal); feeding.
- **Past medical history:**
  - Identify important past or ongoing medical problems that may affect or be affected by the pregnancy;
  - Consider also relevant past gynaecological history (infertility, last cervical smear and result);
  - Past blood transfusion.
- **Drug history** – indication; necessity; change of medication or dose in response to pregnancy; possible teratogenicity; allergies.
- **Family history** – fetal anomalies; genetic conditions; consanguinity; diabetes; hypertension; pre-eclampsia; gestational diabetes; twins.
- **Social history** – occupation; poor social circumstances; smoking; epidemiological risk factors for obstetric problems; misuse of prescribed/recreational drugs.

Antenatal risk factors ('risk scoring')

- Poor obstetric history, e.g. preterm delivery, IUGR, fetal anomaly, stillbirth, abruption
- Extremes of age
- Extremes of weight
- Pre-existing medical conditions, e.g. diabetes, hypertension, psychiatric
- Significant family history
- Smokers
- Drug abusers
- Social deprivation
- Domestic violence

Important points in the gynaecological history

- **Presenting complaint** – main symptom(s) and duration.
- **History of presenting complaint:**
  - Obtain information about the presenting complaint(s) including any tests/treatments;

- Enquire further about other *relevant* gynaecological symptoms (this demonstrates your understanding of potential diagnoses to the examiner). Important 'negative' answers are as important as positive responses;
  - Enquire routinely about cervical smear history and current contraception/contraceptive history (and fertility plans if appropriate) at the end of this part so as not to forget.
- **Systematic enquiry** – cardiovascular; respiratory; gastrointestinal; musculoskeletal; central nervous system.
- **Obstetric history:**
  - This can usually be brief for most gynaecological histories and restricted to number of pregnancies/children, mode of delivery and future fertility plans. However, more detailed exploration may be indicated in some circumstances, e.g. recurrent miscarriage, infertility, urogynaecology.
- **Past medical history:**
  - Enquire about surgical history and past/current medical problems (often also a good time to ask about any medications for particular medical problems);
  - Although 'unexpected' relevant past gynaecological history may arise, try to avoid this by enquiring about any relevant gynaecological history (diagnoses/tests/treatments) in the history of the presenting complaint.
- **Drug history** – including allergies.
- **Family history** – cancer; thrombophilia (if relevant).
- **Social history** – occupation; marital status; tobacco; alcohol; recreational drugs/accommodation (if relevant).

Summary

You may be asked to present a succinct summary to the examiner. Indeed some candidates like to present this to the patient routinely at the end to clarify any issues and to confirm the validity of the history, i.e. the information obtained correctly reflects the patient's true history. This summary should contain the key points within two to three articulate sentences, which will influence further investigation and management. Avoid extraneous information, as the examiner will switch off! This can and should be rehearsed, e.g.

'Mrs X is a 48-year-old nulliparous hairdresser presenting with a 6-month history of non-cyclical pelvic pain that has been refractory to treatment with simple analgesics and the combined oral contraceptive pill. The pain is causing her to take time off work and is affecting her relationship with her family. She has been treated for presumed pelvic inflammatory disease in the past and a recent pelvic ultrasound has been reported as normal.'

Revision checklist for gynaecological histories of presenting complaints

- **Menstrual:**
  - LMP; amount; regularity; duration of menses/cycle length; impact on HRQL; dysmenorrhoea and timing/duration; IMB; PCB; age of menarche; perimenopausal symptoms (as appropriate); symptoms of anaemia;
  - Primary vs secondary amenorrhoea; oligomenorrhoea; menopausal symptoms; weight change; acne; seborrhoea; hirsutism; galactorrhoea.
- **Chronic pelvic pain** – site; onset; character; radiation; periodicity (particularly in relation to the menstrual cycle); duration; relieving/exacerbating factors; associated symptoms; dyspareunia (deep/superficial); GIT/GU systemic enquiry.
- **Vaginal discharge** – colour; odour; amount; itch; cyclical; past history of sexually transmitted infection; diabetes.
- **Urogynaecological** – frequency; volume of voids; thirst; fluid intake; urgency; inability to interrupt flow; dysuria; strangury; haematuria; nocturia; incontinence (stress and provoking factors; urge); prolapse (vaginal discomfort, back pain; feeling of something coming down); bowel function.
- **Fertility:**
  - *Female* – menstrual; reproductive/sexual history (frequency of coitus, libido, dyspareunia); past obstetric history; past medical history (especially history of sexually transmitted infections/abdominal sepsis/ tubal surgery);
  - *Male* – reproductive/sexual history (impotence, ejaculation); past medical history (especially history of sexually transmitted infections/genital operations); social history (environmental and/or occupational exposure to hazardous factors, e.g. smoking, alcohol; occupation (sedentary)).
- **Premenstrual syndrome** – cyclical physical and mental symptoms; headaches; bloating; breast tenderness; change in mood; irritability.
- **Menopausal** – hot flushes; night sweats and insomnia; mood alteration; vaginal dryness; lack of libido; fatigue.

Top tips for patient history taking

1 Ask open-ended questions rather than leading ones and do not use medical terms, e.g. do you have menorrhagia? To speed the history along in a systematic fashion you will probably need to ask more closed, targeted questions to obtain a more detailed description of symptoms in order to formulate a logical history in a coherent fashion. The art is to demonstrate to the examiner that you are giving the patient time to describe in her own words what she perceives to be the problem(s), but are keeping the sequence of questions and responses 'on track'.

2 In a typical obstetric or gynaecological history, it is unlikely that a detailed social history (in contrast to elderly care medicine/psychiatry) or drug history/ systematic enquiry (unlike general medical histories) will be required, but be prepared for this, e.g. domestic violence/drug abuse in an antenatal patient.

3 Concentrate upon the *history of the presenting complaint* and related history rather than trying to be totally 'comprehensive' – trying to cover all aspects of a history leads to loss of focus and confusion, i.e. you end up not being able to 'see the wood for the trees'. This does not mean overlooking other aspects of the history (see above) as these can be taken quite quickly and will gain you marks on the examiner's structured mark sheet. However, discretionary marks and overall marks will be optimized by staying focused upon the *history of the presenting complaint*, thereby producing an individual, tailored history, and understanding the fact that a detailed 'micro-history' of every known obstetric or gynaecological symptom is not required.

4 If the patient appears unsure or uncommunicative check that she has understood your question(s) and ask her if she has anything to add/any questions. Remember, the role player may have been told to be quiet, easily confused, etc.

5 Be aware of the requirements of good history taking (see Table 2.1) so you leave the examiner with a favourable impression of your performance.

TABLE 2.1 Features of good and bad history taking

Feature	Good history	Bad history
Interaction	Engages patient, listens	Disengaged, ignores answers
Questions	Open, unambiguous	Closed, ambiguous
Sequence	Logical, avoid repetition	Illogical, repetition
Emphasis	Focused on presenting complaint	'Scattergun', vague
Information	Relevant, facilitates differential diagnoses	Irrelevant, inability to arrive at differential diagnoses
Time to acquire	Rapid	Slow
Presentation	Succinct, germane	Drawn out, extraneous information

Management

As practising obstetricians and gynaecologists, you spend a large part of your working week formulating what you hope are the most effective, appropriate and acceptable management plans for your patients. It should come as no surprise therefore, that the MRCOG Part 2 clinical examination will seek to assess your competency in this important area. Such stations will ask you to *'outline'* or *'discuss'* or *'explain'* a *'plan of management'* or perhaps *'management options'* with your patient.

The fact you have been invited to attend the clinical examination means that you have already demonstrated to the satisfaction of the RCOG your clinical knowledge *on paper*. The key now is to demonstrate that this knowledge can be put into practice in the 'real' clinical environment. In the written paper you are conveying your knowledge to the examiner reading your manuscript. Although you may be asked direct set questions regarding clinical management (a structured 'viva') in the practical OSCE, it is more common that you will need to convey your knowledge to the examiner via your interaction with the 'patient' sat in front of you. Clearly this sort of station does not just test your ability to devise an appropriate management strategy (often based upon your preceding history); it also tests your skill in communication (see Chapter 3).

Tips on how to approach these two types of clinical management stations are outlined below.

Discuss management with examiner: structured viva

In general, the examiner will ask questions around the management of obstetric or gynaecological problems presenting in an elective (e.g. clinic, inpatient ward, operating theatre) or emergency setting (e.g. labour ward, acute gynaecology unit, A&E department). Make sure you listen carefully to the questions posed and do not rush into an answer without due consideration. It is likely that you have dealt with a similar clinical problem either directly or indirectly and so use this experience to aid you when responding. It is usually quite apparent to the examiner as to which candidates have experience of managing such clinical problems and which need to rely heavily on theoretical 'textbook' recollection of facts.

The beauty of clinical medicine is its diversity and so it is naïve to think that there is always a clear 'right' or 'wrong' answer to managing specific clinical problems. The clinically mature candidate will be able to convey this complexity by considering more than one approach to management whilst avoiding appearing indecisive. A good way of doing this is to outline the available management options, succinctly summarize the pros and cons of each intervention, but then come down on what *you would actually do*. Even if the examiner disagrees with you or your chosen option is not the one advocated on the structured mark sheet, you will score marks by having considered alternative options and your clinical consideration will score overall 'global' discretionary marks. Two examples of this approach are given below.

Example 1: Approach to discussing management options

Would you agree to undertake a hysterectomy in a fit 51-year-old perimenopausal woman with menorrhagia and uterine fibroids who is requesting this intervention despite a benign endometrial biopsy and not having received any medical treatment for the symptom prior to referral?

Consider:
- Pros vs cons:
  - *Pros* – effective treatment; medical treatments more likely to fail in the presence of uterine fibroids; surgical morbidity is likely to be low in an otherwise fit patient;
  - *Cons* – natural menopause imminent; patient may respond well to medical or minimally invasive surgical options; higher surgical morbidity with hysterectomy.
- Patient preferences – impact on her health-related quality of life (HRQL); understanding and awareness of less invasive treatment options and menopause.

Answer – Despite the fact that her bleeding symptoms are likely to resolve soon naturally, in the presence of uterine pathology I would agree to her request if her symptoms are having a significant adverse impact on her HRQL, and she understands the risks associated with surgery and that other effective, simpler treatment options are available.

Example 2: Approach to discussing management options

Would you induce a woman at 36 weeks with an unfavourable cervix who is complaining of pelvic discomfort and difficulty mobilizing attributed to symphysis pubis dysfunction? She has had one previous pregnancy that resulted in an elective caesarean section for a breech presentation and she would like a trial of vaginal delivery this time.

Consider:
- Pros vs cons:
  - *Pros* – SPD may improve more quickly and improve HRQL;
  - *Cons* – increased likelihood of failed IOL and emergency C/S in labour (resulting in longer post-delivery convalescence and prolonged mobility limitations); need for IOL on labour ward as high risk; small risk RDS in preterm neonate; no evidence for benefit of early IOL (or C/S).
- Patient preferences – impact on her HRQL; understanding and awareness of SPD and the potential risks and benefits; conservative treatment options (positional advice; analgesics, physiotherapy, belts).

Answer – Given the facts she has not laboured before, is preterm and has an unfavourable cervix and a uterine scar, on balance quicker resolution of her symptoms (especially if she ends up with an emergency C/S) cannot be guaranteed with induction. I would not advise IOL, but would try to persuade her to delay IOL until at least around 38 weeks if her cervix becomes more favourable. I would explain to her that I believe the risks outweigh any potential benefit, whilst recognizing the impact her symptoms are having on her HRQL, and so would aim to optimize management (analgesics, physiotherapy) and offer her weekly follow-up and additional midwifery support.

Discuss management with patient (role player)

At this situation you must concentrate on the patient, establish a rapport with her and ignore the presence of the examiner. If the station has instructed you to discuss management, i.e. *not* to take a preceding history, then remember to introduce yourself. At all times, however difficult the interaction may become, remain composed and appear professional. Remember that the consultation may not be going well either because you are not communicating well or the role player has been instructed to be uncommunicative or difficult, i.e. she has a set agenda. If the patient is quiet, you should probe for a response by checking if she has understood or has any questions or concerns, requires clarification or has any specific preferences for treatment. Listen and do not interrupt or talk over the patient unless she is being unduly verbose (which she may have been instructed to be!). Whilst you want to convey to the examiner your ability to address all viable management options, you must avoid giving too much information to the patient without pausing for a response from the patient – give information in small 'chunks'. Some candidates like to draw diagrams to aid explanation and patient understanding, but unless this is something you employ in your day-to-day practice (and are good at!), then trying such an approach for the first time in an exam situation may be counterproductive.

Summary of approach to management stations involving a role player

- Introduce yourself
- Explain why you are there
- Remain composed and in control of the consultation – be aware that the role player may have been briefed to be difficult
- Avoid talking too much and concentrate on communication:
  - Break up the consultation by providing information in small 'chunks'
  - Ask if she has any questions, concerns, preferences, or needs you to explain again/provide clarification
  - Use diagrams only if this is part of your usual practice
- Do not interact with the examiner unless instructed to do so

---

Example question and structured mark sheet

OSCE Q – Dysmenorrhoea (History and management)

Candidate's instructions

The patient you are about to see is Cindy Ray, a 23-year-old law student who has been referred because of severe period pain. Her GP found no abnormality on examination but she has been told that she may have something called 'adenomyosis' which has made her very anxious.

Your task is to take a concise, relevant history, address the patient's anxiety and outline the treatment options available.

Marks will be awarded for:

- Taking an appropriate history;
- Ascertaining the reasons for her anxiety and addressing these;
- Discussing likely diagnoses and appropriate management options.

Role player's instructions

You are Cindy Ray, a 23-year-old law student. You are single and have never been sexually active. You have no medical problems of note, but smoke 20 cigarettes a day and drink socially.

Your menstrual cycles are regular and not heavy, but are very painful. The pain is colicky, suprapubic and starts 2 days before your period and generally eases off around day 3 of your period. You have suffered with this pain since menarche aged 16 years. The pain can be so severe as to leave you bed-bound so that you take time off from your studies. You take co-codamol on an ad-hoc basis to combat the pain, but you do not like taking tablets. You do not have any other pain and minimal PMS symptoms.

You are anxious because you have been told you have a disease called adenomyosis, a condition that you do not fully understand but you have read that the condition necessitates a hysterectomy.

Examiner's instructions

Candidate's have 14 minutes to demonstrate the following:

- Ability to take an appropriate history;
- Ability to ascertain the reasons for the patient's anxiety;
- Ability to address the patient's anxiety;
- Ability to discuss likely diagnoses and appropriate management options.

Structured mark sheet

Taking an appropriate history   [4]
Nature, site, pattern (in relation to menstrual cycle) and duration of pain, precipitating/relieving factors, previous treatment, menstrual bleeding history, previous obstetric history, contraceptive/sexual history, relevant medical problems.

0   1   2   3   4

Ascertaining the reasons for her anxiety [2]
- Labelled as having a disease 'adenomyosis' at a young age.
- Uncertainty about the condition and its implications.
- Fear of needing a hysterectomy and its effect on femininity/fertility.

0   1   2

Addressing the reasons for her anxiety and likely diagnoses [4]
- Explanation of diagnosis 'spasmodic primary dysmenorrhoea'.
- Explanation of adenomyosis in simple lay terms and its implications (minimal, can be associated with endometriosis). *'Adenomyosis is a common condition in which tissue that normally lines the uterus (the endometrium) begins to grow inside the muscular outer wall of the uterus which can lead to heavy menstrual bleeding, pain and sometimes an enlargement of the uterus.'*
- General context – spasmodic dysmenorrhoea commoner in nulliparous (young) women (up to 50%), most of whom do not have adenomyosis. May improve after childbirth. Whether adenomyosis or not is irrelevant, as it is the *symptoms* that are treated. Diagnosis is histological (at hysterectomy) but treatment does not necessitate a hysterectomy unless the patient is an older women without future fertility aspirations and who is refractory to other less invasive therapies.
- Individual context – adenomyosis unlikely from symptoms as primary rather than secondary dysmenorrhoea, i.e. relieved with menstrual flow, no pain at other times of cycle (endometriosis which is associated with adenomyosis is unlikely). Classically expect heavy periods and enlarged uterus which she does not have.

0   1   2   3   4

Appropriate management options [6]
- Transabdominal ultrasound (note VI so not transvaginal) may help provide reassurance regarding pelvic anatomy/absence of gynaecological pathology and specifically adenomyosis (although scan has limited accuracy, as does MRI, but if uterus is of normal size and non-suggestive myometrial appearances, then adenomyosis is unlikely).
- General – reassurance, general lifestyle – diet (healthy, oily fish, reduce dairy), exercise, stop smoking. Topical heat (about 39° C).
- Vitamins – B_1, E – 2 days before, first 3 days of menses (RCT suggests benefit, Grade A evidence).

- Simple analgesics – recommend NSAIDs, e.g. mefanamic acid – encourage taking these regularly rather than ad hoc for better pain control and use paracetamol or codeine in between doses. If patient does not like taking tablets, consider rectal suppositories or transdermal preparations.
- First-line hormonal manipulation – COC, try sequential at first, then consider tricycle or continuous.
- Second-line hormonal manipulation – long-acting progestogens (DMPA, Implanon, Mirena).
- Other – transcutaneous electrical nerve stimulation (high frequency stimulation).
- Surgical – third-line, definitive evidence from large RCT that laparoscopic uterosacral nerve ablation is not effective; no strong evidence of benefit and potential for significant morbidity with laparoscopic presacral neurectomy.

0   1   2   3   4   5   6

Global score   **[4]**

0   1   2   3   4

Total: **/20**

3

Communication, counselling and breaking bad news

Since the introduction of the clinical OSCE to MRCOG Part 2 examination with its use of professional role players, it is fair to say that the 'communication and counselling' stations have instilled fear and loathing in equal measure in the prospective part 2 candidate. Candidates recount in vivid detail their traumatic experiences with grief stricken 'patients' or, worse still, encounters with hot-headed 'relatives', apparently incandescent with rage. Although these accounts can shake the most confident candidate, the truth is that with adequate preparation and a modicum of knowledge, these stations can not only be successfully navigated, but can be a fruitful source of easy marks. Hopefully, by the end of this chapter, you will no longer approach these stations with trepidation but embrace them.

Approach to the station

It is possible for the 'bookworm' to pass the written part of the MRCOG Part 2 exam with limited actual clinical time 'spent at the coalface'. However, the clinical OSCE is designed to assess a candidate's clinical experience and so validate their competence to proceed in a career in O&G. OSCE stations requiring 'communication or counselling' are exemplary for assessing competence in dealing with 'real life situations', which cannot simply be 'learnt' from a textbook. In view of this you should concentrate upon showing your counselling skills and not be preoccupied with conveying your knowledge of a subject area. The latter is *not* what is required. You have passed the written part 2 and so your knowledge is taken as read.

That said, there are undoubtedly techniques and approaches to counselling stations that can be practised and 'learnt'. This chapter deals with both generic and specific approaches to communication and counselling situations you may encounter in the exam.

General approach to communications and counselling stations

Recognize the paramount importance of your introduction and manner
- Greet, introduce, gain permission, eye contact
- Speak in a calm and purposeful manner
- Explain why you are here
- Listen attentively
- Sympathetic approach – express condolences, recognize her tragic loss, respect her views
- Do not appear rushed or defensive
- Be honest and do not hesitate to admit what you do not know because maintaining trust matters more than appearing knowledgeable
- Establish a relationship with the patient

Recognize the importance of supportive non-verbal communication
- Maintaining eye contact
- Nodding
- Smiling
- Looks of concern
- Tactile *if* appropriate

Allow patients to express grief/anger
- Do not 'jump in', i.e. listen attentively and do not interrupt, so allowing patients to disclose their feelings, worries and concerns
- Allow silences/pauses
- Offer to come back again if she would like time to herself
- Encourage the patient/family to speak honestly
- Display empathy (verbal and non-verbal) – let the woman know that she is being listened to *and* understood with non-verbal prompts and verbal 'paraphrasing' of what has been said by them (*Examples: 'I can see how angry you are about what happened'; 'So you feel very annoyed that no-one explained the situation to you. …'; 'It must be hard for you with …'*)
- Recognize need to address/acknowledge/validate the emotion expressed (*Examples: 'This must be difficult for you. Can you tell me how you are feeling?' or 'I can see that you are angry'.*)
- Repeat/reinforce information several times and 'offer' to give written information, if possible to back up.

3.1 General communication techniques and skills

Provision of effective and compassionate care requires a good doctor–patient relationship. Such a relationship relies greatly on effective communication. A combination of evidence and theory shows that good communication can improve accuracy of diagnosis, compliance with treatment, clinical outcomes (such as blood pressure and blood glucose levels), a patient's trust in the clinician, patient satisfaction and, last but not least, the clinician's satisfaction. It can also reduce the risk of litigation.

The ability to assess communication skills is the primary advantage an OSCE offers compared to the written MRCOG exam. Effective communication has several components; many of us do most of these naturally. However, careful consideration of the various facets of communication is likely to improve its effectiveness and, of course, enhance the chances of passing the exam! Research evidence has now rejected the traditional opinion that good communication skills are something intrinsic, and little can be done if you are not gifted with such skills. Studies, both within and outside medicine, show that communications skills can be taught, learnt and examined. We provide some didactic guidelines in this chapter.

Greet

'You don't get a second chance to make the first impression.' (Anonymous)

Let's let the evidence speak. A study of 415 patients showed that 91% of them wanted the doctor to address them by name, with 50% preferring the forename, 17% the surname and the rest both names. The same survey found that only 50% of doctors observed this basic expectation of their patients. On the much discussed 'to shake or not to shake' debate, 78% of patients showed a preference to shake hands with their doctor.

So, our evidence-based recommendation is for you to greet the patient with their name (*'Good morning, Mrs Smith'*), introduce yourself (*'I am Dr Patel'*), and offer to shake hands unless you or the patient may be averse to this for cultural or other reasons. Using the patient's forename and surname in an initial greeting will not only set the scene for a good doctor–patient relationship, but also will ensure correct identification of patients, which is an elemental aspect of patient safety.

Names are not just for greeting. Use of a patient's name through the consultation gives her the reassurance that you see her as an individual, and not merely as the next 'case' on the clinic conveyor belt. How much better it is to say, *'Mrs Smith, can you please tell me about any past operations?'*, than

'Next, can you please tell me about any past operations?' Of course, every sentence need not start with the patient's name, but occasional use of her name will add a personal touch.

Define the purpose of the encounter

No meeting should start without an agenda. A medical consultation is no different. Simple explanation of the purpose is likely to put the patient at ease, and give you and the patient a common point to start from. For example, you may start with, *'Your GP has written telling me that you have heavy periods. Is that your main complaint?'* If the patient confirms, then you may go on to set out a joint agenda for the consultation: *'I would like to obtain details of your symptoms, perform an examination, arrange any necessary tests, and discuss possible management options. Are you happy with this plan?'* Such a roadmap is essential to make sure both you and your patient do not get lost during the consultation.

However, very few patients come to a doctor with a single problem. Besides, the reason for referral could have changed. For example, a GP may have referred a patient with heavy periods, but since then an ultrasound arranged to investigate the heavy periods could have shown a large ovarian cyst, which might now be the patient's main complaint. Simply 'letting the patient talk' will elicit such issues. Once you have elicited all the main complaints, negotiate and prioritize the agenda.

Let the patient talk

Research evidence shows that doctors allow patients only 23 seconds to present their story before interrupting! Only 2% of patients feel they get the opportunity to complete their story. This is likely to result in severe restriction of flow of information from the patient, which in turn can compromise the diagnostic process and patient satisfaction. It can also lead to the fateful exam situation in which the OSCE role player asks you, *'What about the 10 cm ovarian cyst that my GP was concerned about?'*, in the final minute of the OSCE station when you are busy rapidly regurgitating treatment options for menorrhagia!

Our recommendation is for you to ask the patient, *'Tell me what is troubling you,'* and then to sit back and listen until she is ready to stop. In the OSCE situation, aim to give the patient at least 90 seconds – research shows that a patient's average opening statement (if uninterrupted) is shorter than 90 seconds. Occasionally a patient may start to throw a number of seemingly unrelated issues at you (my heavy periods, hair loss and right little toe are troubling me). In that situation, it is reasonable to suggest that the patient focuses on one issue at a time, with a promise that you will hear out the others later: *'Tell me about your periods first; you can tell me about the other problems later'* (see below).

Top tip!

All candidates 'talk too much'. Therefore, *consciously* concentrate upon allowing pauses and *not* 'jumping in'. This approach will allow the patient/ relative to express their concerns. Remember that the role player has a scenario and mark sheet to follow and the adoption of such a strategy is likely to give you valuable information and elicit clues as to where the station is leading and where the marks are to be collected.

Listen

Listening is a learnable skill, although a tough one to master. The four elements of good listening are:

- Paying attention;
- Not interrupting;
- Echoing;
- Appropriate non-verbal language.

Let's take these in turn. 'Paying attention' refers to listening with a genuine interest and registering in your mind (and the notes) what the patient has to say, those doctors who have no interest in doing this are probably in the wrong profession. You should switch off your phone, clear your mind of other raging thoughts and get into the frame of mind of: 'I am here to listen to you and help you'. The patient should feel there is no urgency and she has your undivided attention.

'Not interrupting' does not refer to deathly silences which can be discomforting to most patients. It does, however, mean not butting in with questions like, 'How many pads?', 'Any clots?' Encouraging the patient to go on with expressions such as *'Uh-huh'*, *'I see'*, *'Yes'* and *'Go on'* can, of course, be employed.

Echoing refers to the technique that encourages patient to talk and shows empathy.

Example of echoing

Mrs Smith: *The periods are now out of control, doctor. None of the medicines seems to work. I use tampons and towels, and am still getting blood dripping down my legs. I am so fed up with it ...*

Doctor: *Uh-huh.*

Mrs Smith: *... and I have to take 3 or 4 days off work every month. My employer is fed up with me and I am fed up with my periods.*

Doctor: *Both you and your employer are fed up with the situation.* **(echoing)**

Mrs Smith: *Exactly! And my doctor doesn't seem to take it seriously either. I am popping so many tablets, but what good has that done to me?*

Doctor: *Yes, I see ... nothing seems to work ...* **(echoing)**

Mrs Smith: *Well yes, more or less. The pill did work though for a while, but I didn't want to carry on taking it after my mum died of a clot in the chest ...*

Finally, appropriate non-verbal language is the hallmark of good listening skills. Appropriate eye contact, body posture (e.g. arms uncrossed and upper body slightly leaning forward) and use of nods and grunts all let the patient know that you are listening. Remember, it has been said 'non-verbal language speaks louder than verbal language' and if there is discordance between your verbal and non-verbal language, the patient will always believe your non-verbal message.

Question and discuss

The need to let the patient talk and listening must be balanced against your need to obtain a systematic history that allows you to examine various hypotheses regarding potential diagnosis and therapy. After the first 1 or 2 minutes, after the patient has had a chance to tell you her story, you will generally need to guide, quiz, redirect and focus on certain aspects of the story to complete the history. You will need to employ a combination of open (*'Tell me about your periods?'*) and closed questions (*'How many days do you bleed for?'*).

Example of good questioning (continued from scenario above)

Mrs Smith: *Well yes, more or less. The pill did work though for a while, but I didn't want to carry on taking it after my mum died of a clot in the chest ... I didn't want to die like her ... and now this ovarian cyst ... I feel my body is falling apart ... and I am only 27.*

Doctor: *Mrs Smith, I think I understand what brought you here today. Three issues: your heavy periods; the ovarian cyst; and concern about whether what happened to your mother could happen to you.* **(echoing)** *Shall we discuss your periods first? How long have they been a problem?* **(focusing)**

Mrs Smith: *For a good while, doctor.*

Doctor: *How long might that be in months and years?* **(guiding)**

Mrs Smith: *Oh ... I don't know ... maybe 2 years ... maybe 3.*

Doctor: *OK, I see. You haven't kept an accurate record of it, but it sounds like it has been a problem for 2–3 years.*

Mrs Smith: *Yes. And the cyst was diagnosed 2 months ago, and I have got some heaviness on the right side and I think it could be due to the cyst.*

Doctor: *Yes, the heaviness could be related to the cyst. I can see the cyst is worrying you, and we will come back to that and discuss it in detail. However, before we go on to that, shall we finish our discussion on your periods. Tell me please Mrs Smith, how many days do you bleed for when you have your periods?* **(redirecting)**

Provide information and share decision-making

Patient's concerns usually revolve around one of two broad issues:

- Apprehension about the condition (diagnosis, prognosis and cause);
- Anxiety about the medical care (tests and treatment).

Research shows clinicians spend very little time, in some studies just 1 minute, providing information on the illness and options for treatment. An uninformative (from the *patient's view*) consultation can result in a patient visiting her GP seeking further information, non-compliance with tests and treatment, non-attendance at clinics and poor outcome. A robust way to provide information and share decision-making is to use the 'educational sandwich' of ATA – Ask, Tell and Ask.

The first 'Ask' relates to the clinician finding out what the patient's ideas, thoughts and feelings are about the cause, diagnosis, prognosis and treatment of the condition. This step is uniformly ignored by doctors, probably due to its perceived irrelevance. ('With my medical education and MRCOG, I know a great deal about this condition – what would this patient know other than half-truths, misconceptions? Why waste my time exploring these, when I can usefully provide a lecture on this condition?') When planning a route on a map, you need to know the starting location and the destination – if you have no idea of where you are on the map, there is no hope of planning a route to your destination. The same is true with the provision of medical information. Unless you know where your patient 'is' at the outset, your efforts to provide information will not get you very far. How do you put the first 'Ask' of ATA into practice? This is illustrated in the example below.

Example of asking patient for her views about her condition (first 'ask' of ATA)

Doctor: *Mrs Smith, before I explain the ovarian cyst, it would help me to know what you have already learnt about this and what your concerns are.* (An alternative is: *Mrs Smith, people normally have some ideas about ovarian cysts. What are your thoughts?*) **(First 'Ask' of ATA)**

Mrs Smith: *Well, yes, doctor, I know what you are going to say* [tears rolling down the face]. *My aunt had the same. I was fearing the worst.*

Doctor [offering tissues, and leaning forward with concern] *I am sorry to see you upset, Mrs Smith. You mentioned fearing the worst?*

Mrs Smith: *Cancer, doctor, what else?*

Doctor: *That's a frightening thought. I see why you are troubled. Mrs Smith, please don't be troubled. You do not have cancer. What you have is what we call a 'simple cyst'; many women of your age have such cysts. It is a benign condition. We will of course do a blood test to be on the safe side. Of course, if it is causing you pain and you are terribly concerned, we also have the option of removing it.*

Mrs Smith: *Thank heavens, doctor. I haven't slept for days worrying about this. I didn't even tell my husband as I didn't want to worry him. Oh, my poor children, I have been so worried for them.*

Doctor: *I am glad I was able to help you with this, Mrs Smith. Now, let me turn to …*

Example of asking patient for her views about her condition (first 'ask' of ATA) *(continued)*

Whilst cancer was certainly not at the top of the doctor's differential list of items to discuss, it was right at the top of the patient's agenda. If the doctor had not specifically elicited the patient's views about her condition, she may have withheld from sharing it (as was the case with her husband), and the doctor's lectures about CA-125, laparoscopic drainage versus cystectomy, potential complications of laparosocopy, etc would have fallen on deaf ears. Always remember that not all patients are forthcoming with questions and concerns – it is your job to probe if your desire is to help the patient.

The second step of ATA is to tell. Use a variety of approaches. Do *not* use medical jargon; if you must use jargon, then define it. Describe the condition or treatment in words, rephrase your description if it is a particularly complex concept, draw diagrams, use pictures and models, provide written information, use DVDs and, if there is a good information website, direct the patient to it. Clearly, many of these approaches cannot be taken in the OSCE exam, but there is nothing to stop you from drawing a sketch of the gynaecological organs to help the patient (the role player) understand the information you wish to impart. You will generally need to cover the following three broad issues:

- What has happened to me? Is it serious? (**diagnosis and prognosis**)
- Why? (**causation**)
- What will be done to me? And when? (**tests and therapy**)

The final A of ATA refers to asking the patient again to describe what she understands. Understanding relies on transmission (from the doctor), reception (by the patient) and clarification (by both parties). The pragmatic way to assess if the patient has understood is to ask her to summarize the discussion. Two approaches are commonly recommended for this purpose, as illustrated below.

Example of asking patient to summarize a discussion (final A of ATA sandwich)

Approach 1

Doctor: *When you go home, your husband will probably ask you about the discussions we have had today. Please tell me what you will tell him? This will help me understand if I have explained the various issues sufficiently.*

Approach 2

Doctor: *I would like to make sure I have explained the issues clearly. Please tell me what you heard so that I can check to see if I have explained the issues adequately.*

A simple 'Is it OK?' is simply not OK. The questions, '*Is there anything else you would like me to tell you?*' and '*Is there any aspect you would like me to go over again?*,' should complement the approaches above, and not replace them!

At the completion of the visit, the clinician can summarize the agreed plans and discuss the next steps (next appointment, referral for tests or therapy elsewhere). There is a view held by some experts that patients regress into a state of juvenile dependence, hoping that the doctor will know what's wrong with them, perhaps with the help of some tests; furthermore, there is the view that there is a single best treatment for most conditions. This, unfortunately, is the exception in medicine. Good communication skills are essential in bridging the many gaps between clinicians and patients, and patients' stories and clinician's history records, so that good quality care can be provided.

Summary of general approach to communication and counselling stations

- Greet
- Define the purpose of the encounter
- Let the patient talk
- Listen
- Question and discuss
- Provide information and share decision-making

3.2 Difficult communication situations

Certain situations can be difficult for the patient, doctor or both. However, there are often tried and tested approaches that can be used to enhance the outcomes in such situations. In this section, we take you through the most important ones and provide practical help, including phrases and sentences you can use to help your patient, help yourself and, of course, help you pass your OSCE exam! You need to have primed yourself with the contents of Chapter 2 and section 3.1 to get the most out of this section.

Giving bad news

Breaking bad news is difficult and as a clinician you have to develop skills to connect and communicate effectively with your patients. Bad news and tragic outcomes can be very disturbing for all concerned and evoke a range of emotions. It is acceptable to empathize with someone's difficult situation, sadness, shock, tragedy, loss. Remember that this is a professional examination and these stations are an opportunity for the RCOG to assess your competence in dealing with 'real life situations' which cannot be 'learnt' from a textbook. We recommend the following steps for 'good' delivery of bad news.

Step 1: Prepare

Preparation is the key. In your OSCE, take your time to *read and understand* the information provided on the station notice board and prepare your approach before entering the exam cubicle and facing the patient (the role player). In real practice, pore over the notes, discuss the case with your senior colleagues, nurses and other relevant professionals, and find out as much as possible about the condition (particularly prognosis, therapy and support) before meeting the patient. Choose a quiet place where you are unlikely to be interrupted. Turn your phone off. Decide whether you wish to have a nurse or another person present.

Step 2: Give a warning note (or two)

A patient needs to be ready to receive the bad news. For example, the following discourse is unlikely to register fully in the mind of a patient: 'Good Morning, Mrs Taylor. I am afraid the ultrasound shows the baby has passed away'. This is referred to as 'dropping the bomb' – warning notes avoid this situation. We show how warning notes are used in two different situations to prepare the patient.

Examples of giving warning notes

Situation 1

You are the senior registrar and an experienced obstetric scanner. You have been called in to see a term woman after your registrar has been unable to find the fetal heart on ultrasound. Your scanning shows the absence of a fetal heart – the diagnosis is stillbirth.

Doctor: *Mrs Taylor, I am unable to see any movements of the baby on the scan.* **(warning note 1)**

Doctor: *… and I am unable to see the baby's heart beat.* **(warning note 2)**

Mrs Taylor: *Oh my God, Oh my God, is the baby dead?*

Doctor: *I am really sorry to give you this news … Yes, the baby has died.*

Situation 2

You are about to give the information that an endometrial biopsy from a woman with PMB has shown endometrial cancer.

Doctor: *Mrs Davis, I would like to discuss the findings of the biopsy you had last week, if that is OK with you.*

Mrs Davis: *Go right ahead doctor, I have been anxious to find out. Was it a polyp?*

Doctor: *We were hoping it would be just a polyp … but I am afraid the news is worse than that.* **(warning note 1)**

Doctor: *Some of the cells looked abnormal under the microscope.* **(warning note 2)**

Mrs Davis: *Abnormal?*

Doctor: *Yes, the biopsy shows it is in fact cancer of the lining of the womb.*

Mrs David: *You said it is cancer?*

Doctor: *Yes, it is cancer.* **(repetition)**

Mrs Davis: *Oh my God, I am going to die.*

Doctor: *Is that how it sounds … like it is all over … there is no hope?* **(echoing)**

Patient: *What can I hope with cancer?*

Doctor: *Well, many people with cancer can be successfully treated. People have different understanding of the word cancer. Can you please bear to tell me what it means to you?* **(First 'Ask' for ATA**, see above)

> **Examples of giving warning notes** *(continued)*
>
> [Once the doctor has established an understanding of Mrs Davis' ideas, concerns and expectations (ICE) regarding cancer and cancer treatment, they are in a position to provide effective counselling.]

Step 3: Play it straight

Once the warning note(s) has been given, the patient will not only be ready, but also very likely anxious, to know the finding. After giving the warning note(s), it is cruel to meander around the issue with trivialities such as, 'Did you find parking OK?' or 'The weather is changing fast, isn't it?', or even with relevant but perhaps less pressing issues such as, 'Tell me, how is the pain now?' or 'Do you have anyone to look after you at home?' The rule is that after the warning note, the bad news needs to be given. It is important to use non-technical language (e.g. cancer not neoplasm) and to be honest (cancer and not 'a bit of a growth'). Whilst it is important to break the bad news with appropriate affect, there is no need to go into 'undertaker mode' with exaggerated gloominess and hopelessness.

Step 4: Be responsive and repeat as often as necessary

As receiving bad news can often induce a degree of temporary mental paralysis, be ready to find out how much has been absorbed by patient, and what would be usefully repeated by you. You have to tell a little, pause, observe the reaction and tell a little bit more or repeat as necessary. You may want to provide written information, and must always leave the patient with an avenue to get support (from you, the team or an emergency telephone line).

Step 5: Give (appropriate) hope

Even in the bleakest situations, there are reasons for hope. For example, someone with a terminal cancer, may find hope in the possibility of a period of remission, or the prospect of a pain-free peaceful death. Never get into the game of giving precise prognostications about survival – whatever you say is likely to be wrong! An approach to handling a survival question is illustrated below.

Example of handling a survival question

Mrs Davis has terminal cancer. You have offered palliative care.

Mrs Davis: *Doctor, how long have I got?*

Doctor: *Mrs Davis, I am sorry. The trouble is none of us knows. It depends on how you respond to the treatment and many other issues.*

Mrs Davis: *Doctor, will I be here for Christmas?*

Doctor: *I realize the uncertainty must be terrible for you. Mrs Davis, I am really sorry, but there is no way of predicting the future. However, what I can do is to put forward the symptoms and signs that you could look for to see if you are deteriorating. Would it help if I told you what they are?*

Mrs Davis: *Yes, doctor. I think that would help ... please go ahead.*

How you give bad news really matters to the patient. Attending a course on this and sitting in with bereavement and cancer counsellors are important ways to acquire the necessary skills.

Top tip: Do's and don'ts of breaking bad news

Do
- Have the facts to hand
- Check if the patient wants anyone else present
- Clarify what the patient knows or suspects
- Be prepared to follow the patient's agenda
- Observe and acknowledge the patient's emotional reactions
- Check patient's understanding of what you are saying

Don't
- Give too much information at one time
- Give inappropriate reassurance
- Answer questions unless you have the facts to hand
- Hurry the consultation
- Use euphemisms
- Stop emotional expressions from the patient
- Agree to relative's request to withhold information from the patient

The angry patient or relative

Overall, the aim is to resolve conflict positively. In reality you would pay attention to the environment, e.g. move the patient to a quiet area as the angry patient with an audience will be less likely to accept your point of view. However, in the OSCE scenario such insight cannot be demonstrated, but the following techniques must be deployed and demonstrated to the examiner.

Top tip: Respect

The use of the person's name in a respectful way (i.e. not forename) in your reply can ease the situation, i.e. Mr Smith, Mrs Jones.

The common causes for anger in a patient include delayed appointments, missed diagnosis, lack of therapeutic success and several forms of miscommunications. The anger may be directed at you, a colleague or an establishment.

An angry patient often triggers the doctor's own fight-or-flight responses, and a host of other responses, including annoyance and exasperation. However, an appropriate approach can often defuse the anger and re-establish effective communication with the patient. Many clinicians adopt the approach of disregarding the anger and 'acting normal' or simply attempting to placate the patient without an attempt at understanding the underlying cause of anger – both of these strategies are likely to aggravate the patient, leading to further deterioration of the situation. We show a constructive approach to managing an angry patient.

Step 1: Listen: 'Get curious; not furious'

Let the patient speak her mind without interruption. The fundamental rule is that the patient's story needs to be heard. Your genuine 'curiosity' about what has angered the patient is the first step in resolving the situation. By staying curious, you can avoid being defensive and expressing opinions before the patient finishes her story. You should aim to find out the specifics of the story by encouraging the patient to give the details. You need to remain calm and establish eye contact, get the patient to sit down and try to adopt a similar posture to the patient (mirroring) without an aggressive pose.

Example of good practice in getting a patient to explain why she is angry

Mrs Patel is angry that she spent over an hour trying to park in the hospital car park, and now has been told off by the receptionist for being late.

Mrs Patel: *Damn it! This place is not here to serve patients! It's crazy that one has pay for the car park, and still wait for an hour to find a spot to put your car.*

Doctor: *Sorry to hear that Mrs Patel … I see you had a tough time trying to find a spot to park.* **(echoing)** *Having to wait for an hour for a parking spot is a long time. I can see how that would be frustrating.* **(empathizing)**

Mrs Patel: *… and the receptionist was rude. It seems rudeness is an attribute required to work in this place.*

Doctor: *I am sorry to hear that. Please tell me more about what the receptionist said to you.* (maintaining **curiosity**)

(Mrs Patel describes the events)

Step 2: Empathize and deal with emotions

Empathy is defined as the identification with and understanding of another's situation, feelings, thoughts and motives. By displaying understanding and concern you can help the person feel understood. Listening and 'putting yourself in another's shoes' are approaches that lead to empathy. One extremely useful and effective technique is 'echoing', i.e. paraphrasing the patient's comments to convey that you have heard and are seeking to understand. All these approaches are illustrated below.

It is important to encourage expression of feelings – *emotions*. Concentrate upon dealing with the patient's feelings and avoid rationalizing. Acknowledge and validate the emotion so the angry patient feels that you are listening to her, e.g. '*You seem very angry?*' Demonstrate your understanding: '*I can see how angry you are about what happened*' and '*It must be hard for you*'.

Top tip!

Concentrate upon dealing with the person's feelings and avoid rationalizing as this approach is likely to inflame the situation, i.e. an 'explanation' is unlikely to be taken in and may come across as an excuse. It is important to encourage expression of feelings. Attempting to defuse anger, ignoring it or, worse still, countering it with your own anger will be counterproductive. Acknowledging the patient's right to be angry is the best approach as it will begin the healing process and solidify the clinical relationship.

Step 3: Take an action (if appropriate)

If you are at fault, you may offer an apology. Aim to be an advocate for the patient where possible (even if you are at fault!). Point the patient in the direction of resources, e.g. *'Would it help if I put you in touch with the Patient Advisory Liaison Service?'* or *'Please tell me if you wish to make a complaint – I can help you with this'*. Ironically, a genuine offer of help often results in the patient not pursuing a formal complaint.

The above three steps apply as long as the patient is angry but not abusive. With a physically abusive patient, you should remove yourself from the scene and call for help. There is no reason for you to tolerate or try to empathize with a verbally abusive patient – the correct approach is to terminate the consultation, but with an offer to help: *'Mrs Patel, I really want to listen and understand your concern, but I can't do that if you continue to use inappropriate language'*.

Disagreement between patient and doctor

Disagreements between patients and doctors regarding precise diagnosis and therapy, and occasionally prognosis, are common. Such disagreements can result in non-compliance with tests, medications and appointments, a search for second opinion(s) and non-conventional therapies and, on occasion, even complaints. The abundance of health information (and mis-information) from magazines, the Internet and medical guidelines often results in patients forming ideas about diagnosis and treatment before they step into a doctor's office. How should you deal with these? We illustrate some principles with the example below.

Example of dealing with disagreement between doctor and patient

Mr and Mrs Khan seek a consultation with you for a 4-year history of infertility. The clinical history (of infrequent periods), androgenic hormone profile and typical ultrasound appearances indicate PCOS. You suggest clomiphene treatment after semen analysis and tubal assessment. However, Mrs Khan pulls a magazine from her handbag, and shows you a story about a woman who had healthy twins following treatment with herbal medicine and acupuncture. There are three potential approaches you can take: we recommend the last of these three!

Approach 1
This is nonsense! Chinese medicine and acupuncture will not correct anovulation. Don't waste your time and money on these please, Mrs Khan.

Approach 2
Yes … why not? Let's find a local herbalist for you.

Approach 3
Can I make a copy of this article? I would like to look into the merits of this article to see if there is anything in it that can help you. I am glad that you are looking into these issues. However, I must confess that herbal medicine and acupuncture are not recognized treatments for women who do not ovulate. So, the likelihood is that the woman in this magazine article got lucky, and her pregnancy may be unrelated to the treatment she received.

Outright rejection of a patient's suggestion (as in Approach 1) is likely to set you and your patient on a war path where there will be little common ground. She may seek to go to a doctor who agrees with her ideas about how she should be treated, or simply go to the herbalist, rejecting your advice. Approach 2 is unethical (unless you yourself believe in her approach, in which case there is no disagreement) as you should maintain your professional integrity and role as the patient's advocate, acting in her best interest. Approach 3 offers the middle-way. However, what if she still disagrees with you? Read on.

Mrs Khan: *I hear you doctor, but I have so many friends who have now benefited from herbal medicine and acupuncture.*

Doctor: *I understand, Mrs Khan. Could I please find out more about what you know about these therapies, and how you feel they may help you. Your thoughts may help me in helping you.* **(eliciting ICE – ideas, concerns and expectations)**

Example of dealing with disagreement between doctor and patient *(continued)*

Mrs Khan: *Thank you, doctor. I think the herbs and acupuncture will readjust my hormone levels; that is bound to help my ovaries to release eggs, don't you agree? In fact, I have seen a herbalist already, who has recommended a course of treatment. I hope to start this treatment next week, but I wanted to chat to you before that.*

Doctor: *OK, Mrs Khan, I see that you have really looked into this approach, and have a lot of faith in it. From scientific data, I have the view that the best treatment for you is clomiphene. I am anxious for you to start clomiphene sooner rather than later, as your advancing age is an important factor in reducing your fertility prospects. So, let me suggest a middle-way: You try herbal medicine for 3 months, and if there is no joy, we will start clomiphene?*

Mrs Khan: *Great! I am very happy with that plan doctor.*

When a patient has firm views, you can gently challenge these and try to negotiate a course of action. However, there is no point in trying or coerce the patient into accepting something she does not wish. A patient has the right to autonomy and self-determination. However, if the patient chooses a path that is harmful to her, then you should communicate the facts firmly, but empathetically. In the end you may 'agree to disagree' and such consultations should be carefully documented. Recommending a second opinion in such situations is considered good practice. When a patient's suggestions are unlikely to harm her, then it is reasonable to make concessions and find a middle-way (as in the example above).

Disclosing medical errors and complications

Research shows that medical errors, complications and 'near misses' are common. Medical defence lawyers have encouraged generations of clinicians not to get involved in disclosing medical errors and certainly not offering apologies for fear of litigation. However, the General Medical Council is clear on this issue: the recommendation is that after an adverse event a full and honest explanation and an apology, if appropriate, should be provided routinely. There are several good reasons for this. There is now good evidence that disclosure of medical errors can in fact reduce the overall rates of litigation! However, the more important reason is that it helps the patient to handle and to come to terms with the complication. How do you achieve this difficult task? As often clichéd, sorry is often the hardest word to say. We take you through this step by step.

Step 1: Prepare yourself

Many organizations have a 'disclosure policy', and you should familiarize yourself with this, and aim to work within the framework provided by such policies. For example, it may be necessary to involve a risk or clinical governance manager before disclosure about serious events that took place. Find out as much as you can about the complications and their implications, and the specific circumstances of the error. Find out what steps need to be taken if the patient is still at risk from the error or complication.

Step 2: Prepare the patient

Start with warning notes (see p. 39), e.g.:

- *'I am afraid I have some upsetting news for you.'* (**warning note 1**)
- *'There was a complication at the time of the surgery.'* (**warning note 2**)
- *'We caused an injury to the ureter, the tube that connects your kidney to the bladder, during the surgery.'* (**communication of the error**)

Step 3: Communicate the error

This needs to be done with honesty and be limited to the information truly known at that point in time. As unpleasant as it may be for the doctor and patient, uncertainties will need to be shared. Unnecessary speculation should be avoided.

Step 4: Apologise, if that is the correct response

It is perfectly acceptable to say *'I am sorry'*. This statement does not necessarily reflect an admission of liability – it can also be an empathetic response to the patient's predicament.

Disclosure can of course result in litigation whether 'I am sorry' is said or not. Furthermore, non-disclosure itself is now considered a primary reason for litigation. Thus, a full disclosure, with an apology if necessary, is the proper approach to take as it is likely to achieve the primary objective of helping the patient deal with the complication and its consequences.

Step 5: Give evidence that you are taking steps

Studies show that patients who have suffered complications seek reassurance that steps will be taken to minimize the occurrence of such complications. Often, it is sufficient to explain that the matter will be investigated and appropriate changes made. Offer to keep the patient informed.

To err is human. Errors and complications will always remain part of clinical medicine, no matter how hard we try to avoid them. An honest approach is the best way when such events occur.

Summary of approach to specific communication and counselling stations

Giving bad news
- Prepare
- Give a warning note (or two)
- Play it straight
- Be responsive and repeat as often as necessary
- Give (appropriate) hope

Angry patient
- 'Get curious, not furious'
- Empathize and deal with emotions
- Take action (if appropriate)

Disagreement between patient and doctor
- Challenge (gently but firmly)
- Negotiate but avoid coercion
- Compromise if appropriate
- Consideration of seeking a second opinion in such situations is good practice

---

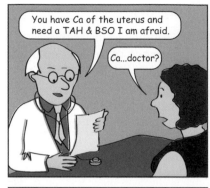
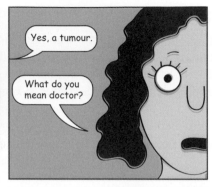
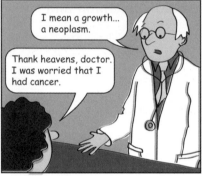
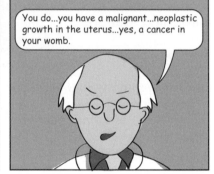

3.3 Better words and phrases for lay communication

'It is remarkably easy not to say what you mean.' (Appleton, *BMJ* 1994)

Research shows that patients are often confused by their doctor's language. For example, a study found that only 60% of cancer patients understood that the term 'metastasis' meant cancer was spreading and only around half knew the term 'remission' meant there was no detectable sign of cancer. One way to improve your chances of helping a patient understand what you are telling her is to choose your words and phrases carefully. How would you explain to a woman the terms 'choroid plexus cysts' or 'trophoblastic disease'? 'Jargon Buster' over the next few pages will benefit your patients and improve your chances in the OSCE.

If you think of a word or phase that you find particularly troublesome to explain to your patient, we suggest you track down a patient information leaflet on the subject of that word or phrase, and in it you are likely to find a way of expressing the word or phrase in plain English.

Jargon buster

Jargon	Lay explanation
Abruption	A (often sudden) breaking off of the afterbirth from the womb
Adenomyosis	Womb thickening due to tissues which should only be found in the inner lining of the womb being present in the actual muscle of the womb
AFP (alpha-fetoprotein)	A blood protein that helps to estimate the chance of conditions like Down syndrome
Amniocentesis	A specialized test that involves taking a sample of fluid from the womb with a needle, and examining it in the laboratory to see whether the baby has any serious conditions. It is a diagnostic test, which means that it can tell with almost certainty whether or not the baby has got a particular condition
Anembryonic pregnancy	Empty pregnancy sac
Anencepahly	A condition in which the brain and skull of the baby do not form
Anterior colporrhaphy	An operation to correct the bulging of the bladder into the vagina
Antiphospholipid syndrome	A disorder of the immune system in which there can be clotting within arteries or veins, miscarriages and a variety of other problems, some life-threatening
Biophysical profile (BPP) scoring	An ultrasound test to assess the condition of the baby. The BPP measures the baby's heart rate, muscle tone, movement, breathing, and the amount of amniotic fluid around the baby
Cerebral palsy	A group of conditions in which the baby's brain is damaged before, during or after birth. Affected children can have various disabilities, including problems with thinking, speech, movement, coordination and learning
Choriocarcinoma	Cancer of the afterbirth (placental) tissues
Choroid plexus cyst	Collection of fluid in cysts in the part of the brain which makes the fluid that cushions the brain and spinal cord. This is a normal ultrasound finding in most women. In some instances, it can indicate a chromosomal (see Chromosomes below) condition in the baby, with an extra copy of chromosome 18

Jargon buster *(continued)*

Jargon	Lay explanation
Chorionic villus sampling	A specialized test that involves taking a small piece of afterbirth tissue from the womb with a needle, and examining it in the laboratory to see whether the baby has any serious conditions. It is a diagnostic test, which means that it can tell with almost certainty whether or not the baby has got a particular condition
CIN (cervical carcinoma in situ)	A condition in which the neck of the womb (cervix) has cells that are not normal – these cells have a chance of becoming cancer, so the neck of the womb needs to be monitored or treated
Colposcopy	A detailed examination of the neck of the womb with an instrument which provides magnified views
Chromosomes	Thread-like structures in the cells that are the 'building blocks of life', containing the genes; there are 46 of them in humans
Colposuspension	An operation to treat urinary leakage, by providing special support to the bladder and the tube that connects the bladder to the outside (urethra)
CTG	A test that assesses the baby's condition by recording the baby's heart rate. It also records the contractions of the womb
Cytology	Laboratory examination of cells (e.g. from the neck of the womb)
Cystoscopy	An examination of the bladder and the passageway that takes urine from the bladder to the outside (urethra) with a special telescope-like instrument
Cystic fibrosis	An inherited condition in which the body produces thick sticky mucus that damages lungs and other organs
Cystocoele	A condition in which the bladder bulges into or through the vagina
Cystourethrocoele	A condition in which the bladder and the passageway that takes urine from the bladder to the outside bulge through the vagina
Deep venous thrombosis	A blood clot forming in a large vein, like the veins in the leg or thigh. The blood clot can break off and travel in the circulation, and can become lodged in the brain, lungs, heart or other area, severely damaging that organ

Jargon buster *(continued)*

Jargon	Lay explanation
Diagphramatic hernia	A birth defect in which there is a hole in the diaphragm, the muscle that separates the chest from the tummy (abdomen); this hole allows slipping of the bowel into the chest, causing distress with breathing
Down's syndrome	A condition that is most commonly caused by an extra copy of chromosome 21 (see Chromosomes above), in which the child has a typical facial appearance, learning difficulties as well as other complications such as heart defect
Dyskaryosis	A smear finding in which there are changes in the appearance of the cells that cover the neck of the womb (cervix). It is not cancer, but in some women it can become cancer over a period of time; thus it requires monitoring or treatment
Electrocardiogram (ECG)	A heart trace
Eclampsia A Greek word meaning 'bolt from the blue'.	It is a serious complication of pregnancy characterized by convulsions or fits. It is associated with high blood pressure and protein in the urine (pre-eclampsia)
Echocardiogram	An ultrasound test of the heart that gives information about any defects, such as holes in the heart, as well as the pumping action of the heart
Edwards syndrome	A condition that is caused by an extra copy of chromosome 18 (see Chromosomes above); very few babies survive this condition; when they survive, they can have serious physical and learning disabilities
Epidural	Injection of pain-killing and anaesthetic drugs through a catheter ('a tube') placed in the small of the back, going into the space outside the coverings that surround the spinal cord
Embryo	A life at very early stages of development. Note: 'embryo' often refers to life from fertilization to 8 weeks; after 8 weeks, the term 'fetus' is often used
Endometrium	The inner lining of the womb
Endometrial polyp	A 'finger-like projection' or 'fleshy swelling' in the inner lining of the womb
Endometriosis	A condition in which tissues that normally line the womb (endometrium) are found elsewhere, like internal lining of the abdomen (tummy)

Jargon buster *(continued)*

Jargon	Lay explanation
Enterocoele	A condition in which the bowels bulge into or through the vagina
Episiotomy	A surgical cut in the vagina and surrounding skin to make room for the vaginal delivery of a baby
Fibroids	A fibroid is a benign ('non-cancerous') growth in the womb. It can occur anywhere in the womb, and can vary from pea-sized to the size of a melon
Gastroschisis	A condition in which the intestines and sometimes other organs bulge through a hole in the fetal abdomen (tummy)
Group B streptococcus (GBS)	A bacterial infection that can be passed to a baby during delivery. It can cause severe infection in a newborn baby. However, it is not a sexually-transmitted infection, and outside pregnancy many women have the bacteria without it causing any harm to them
Genes	Genes are 'building blocks of life' which code for human characteristics
Human chorionic gonadotrophin (hCG)	A 'pregnancy hormone' that is produced by the afterbirth tissues (placenta)
Histology	Assessment of tissues in the laboratory with a microscope
HPV screening	Testing for viruses that can cause abnormal cells which, in turn, can lead to cancer in the neck of the womb (if left untreated)
Hystero-contrast-sonography (HyCoSy)	An ultrasound test to check whether the fallopian tubes are blocked or open, by putting a special dye through a catheter ('plastic tube') placed in the womb
Hysterosalpingography (HSG)	An X-ray test to check whether the fallopian tubes are blocked or open, by putting a special dye through a catheter ('plastic tube') placed in the womb
Hysterosocopy	A test to look inside the womb using a narrow tube-like telescope
Hydrosalpinx	A blocked, dilated, fluid-filled fallopian tube, usually caused by a previous tubal infection
Hydrophic fetus	An abnormal accumulation of fluid in the baby, e.g. in the lungs, around the heart and in the abdomen
ICSI	ICSI is a technique sometimes used in IVF (see IVF below) in which one sperm is injected directly into one egg in order to fertilize it

Jargon buster *(continued)*

Jargon	Lay explanation
IVF	An assisted reproductive technique in which the ovaries are stimulated with drugs to produce a large number of eggs which are collected from the ovaries with a needle, to be inseminated with the partner's sperm in a test-tube to create embryos which are then transferred into the woman's womb to give the couple a chance of pregnancy
Karyotype	The complete set of chromosomes (see Chromosomes above) inside the nucleus of a cell
Laparoscopy	A keyhole operation to look inside the abdomen and pelvis using a narrow tube-like telescope
Laparotomy	A surgical incision on the abdomen to look and treat inside the abdomen or pelvis
Lichen sclerosis	A condition in which the skin around the vagina (vulva) becomes thin, white, shiny and often itchy; the condition is important as it has a small chance of giving rise to cancer
LLETZ (large loop excision of the transformation zone); loop cone biopsy	An operation to remove a small piece of the neck of the womb with the aim of removing abnormal cells from the neck of the womb
Meconium	The green amniotic fluid resulting from the baby opening its bowel while inside the mother's womb
Metastasis	Transfer of cancer from one organ to another
Neural tube defects	Serious birth defects in which the brain, spinal cord, or their coverings do not develop completely
Nuchal translucency	A collection of fluid under the skin at the back of a baby's neck, measured with an ultrasound scan at 10–14 weeks' gestation. It is a screening test for Down syndrome
Obstetric cholestasis (cholestasis of pregnancy or intrahepatic cholestasis of pregnancy)	A condition of the mother's liver that is thought to be due to the liver over-responding to pregnancy hormones. It causes itchiness and carries risks to the mother and baby
Ovum	Egg (from the ovary)
Placenta praevia	A pregnancy complication in which the afterbirth (placenta) has attached to the wall of the womb close to or covering the neck of the womb (cervix)
Polyp	(See Endometrial polyp above)
Polypectomy	Removal of a polyp (see Endometrial polyp above)

Jargon buster *(continued)*

Jargon	Lay explanation
Pre-eclampsia	Pre-eclampsia is a serious condition of pregnancy. It is associated with high blood pressure and protein in the urine, and can cause complications such as convulsions and damage to organs such as the liver, kidneys and lungs
Proteinuria	Passing protein in the urine
Pulmonary embolism	Simplest explanation: A serious condition in which there are blood clots in the lungs Detailed explanation: A serious condition in which there is a blockage in the blood vessels in the lungs with blood clots; these blood clots often come from dislodged blood clots from other blood vessels such as the veins in the legs
Rectocoele	A condition in which the rectum bulges into or through the vagina
Remission	A state of absence of disease
Respiratory distress syndrome (neonatal)	A breathing disorder in a newborn baby that can sometimes cause serious distress and harm to the baby
Salpingectomy	Removal of fallopian tube(s), often through key-hole surgery
Septicaemia	Blood poisoning with bacterial infection
Smear test	A simple test to collect cells from the neck of the womb (cervix); these cells are tested in the laboratory to see if they have a risk of becoming cancerous
Shoulder dystocia	A serious condition in which the baby's shoulder gets stuck behind the mother's pelvic bone, soon after delivery of the baby's head
Spinal anaesthesia	Injection of pain-killing and anaesthetic drugs through a catheter ('a tube') placed in the small of the back, going into the space outside the spinal cord
Spina bifida	(See Neural tube defect above.) This is the most common neural tube defect, in which the spine does not close properly during early pregnancy development
Stillbirth	Death of a baby inside the womb
Thrombophilia	A range of conditions that results in an individual having 'sticky blood', and thus an increased risk of clots forming in blood vessels, as well as other complications such as miscarriages

Jargon buster *(continued)*

Jargon	Lay explanation
Trophoblastic disease, molar pregnancy, hydatifiform mole	Abnormal overgrowth of the afterbirth (see also Choriocarcinoma above)
TVT (tension-free vaginal tape)	A TVT operation is performed to help women with incontinence. Two small cuts are made on the lower part of the tummy and another small cut in the vagina. A special tape is then passed through these cuts to form a sling around the tube that lets urine flow out of the bladder (urethra)
Umbilical Doppler test	An ultrasound test of blood flow through the umbilical cord of the baby. The test gives information on the baby's well-being, which often helps us decide on the timing of delivery of the baby
Urodynamic testing	A test performed for a detailed understanding of the way the bladder functions by evaluating urine flow, pressure and volume. A small catheter (tube) will be passed into the bladder via the urethra ('the pipe that empties urine from the bladder to the outside'), to help us perform this test
Uterine artery Doppler test	An ultrasound test of blood flow through the main blood vessels of the womb. The test gives information on the risks of a pregnant woman developing blood pressure complications ('pre-eclampsia') or having a poorly nourished ('growth restricted') baby

Example question and structured mark sheet

OSCE Q – Neural tube defect (encephalocoele) (Breaking bad news)

Candidate's instructions

You have been asked to see Mrs Simms, who had a high-resolution ultrasound scan following a very high level of AFP at serum screening. The experienced ultrasonographer who scanned her has told you that she found a large cystic paracranial mass, consistent with an encephalocoele. Mrs Simms is not aware of the diagnosis yet.

You are expected to break the news to Mrs Simms and to counsel her. You will have an examiner observing your consultation.

Marks will be awarded for:

- Explaining the diagnosis;
- Appropriately counselling Mrs Simms about the options;
- Answering Mrs Simms' queries with sympathy and tact.

Role player's instructions

You are Mrs Simms. You have just had an ultrasound scan following a very high level of AFP at serum screening. The ultrasonographer who scanned you has told you nothing but has sent you to see the obstetrician to discuss the scan result.

The candidate (obstetrician) is required to explain the scan result to you and to break bad news.

Questions you should ask during the consultation:

1. Is this due to my smoking? I knew I should have given up.
2. Are you sure about this diagnosis?
3. With a cyst outside the brain, would vaginal delivery still be possible?
4. Is this genetic? Will I get this again?

Examiner's instructions

Candidates have 14 minutes to demonstrate the following:

- Ability to explain the diagnosis in a clear manner.
- Ability appropriately to counsel the patient and discuss management options.
- Ability to communicate and break bad news.
- *Ability to answer the patient's queries with sympathy and tact.*

Structured mark sheet

Basics [4]
- Introduction/eye contact/body language.
- Avoidance of medical jargon.
- Information in small doses; repetition of important information; periodical check for understanding.
- Non-directive and sympathetic counselling.
- Allow patient to talk, express concern/shock, ask questions.

0   1   2   3   4

Diagnosis and management [6]
- Give a warning shot: '*I am afraid the ultrasound has shown a serious finding*'.
- Communicate finding without delay: '*The ultrasound shows brain tissues have escaped through a hole in the skull to form a cyst*'.
- Discuss the prognosis: '*Difficult to predict the outcome – in terms of survival as well as development. Likely to survive, but with disability*' (isolated meningocele – good prognosis; microcephaly associated with brain herniation – very poor prognosis).
- Offer TOP (timing of TOP unlimited by the Abortion Act 1991, Clause E):
  - If accepted, discuss details of TOP (intracardiac K; medical TOP – mefipristone and misoprostol); may need surgical evacuation of RPOC; pain relief;
  - If TOP declined: routine antenatal care; expect vaginal delivery (but be aware of risk of caesarean section); appointment with paediatric neurologist.

0   1   2   3   4   5   6

Role player questions [4]

1. 'Is this due to my smoking? I knew I should have given up.' – No; not related to anything you have or have not done.
2. 'Are you sure about this diagnosis?' – Yes; however, I would be very happy to arrange a second opinion.
3. 'With a cyst outside the brain, would vaginal delivery still be possible?' – In most cases, vaginal delivery is possible – slightly increased risk of caesarean.
4. 'Is this genetic? Will I get this again?' – It may be associated with a genetic problem in this fetus, but that does not mean you or your partner have a genetic condition which would result in recurrent neural tube defects. However, there is an increased risk of NTDs in the future (1/30); thus, high dose folate and high resolution USS in future pregnancies.

0   1   2   3   4

Support, follow-up and closing up [3]

- Summarize.
- Action plan and timelines.
- Information about access to services (including support groups).
- Counselling.
- Offer of further appointments and second opinion.
- Written literature.

0   1   2   3

Role player assessment [3]

Satisfaction with the consultation.

0   1   2   3

Total: **/20**

4 Results interpretation and management

You may arrive at a station and be presented with a test result or series of test results to analyze and interpret. Such stations not only examine your ability to extract information from diagnostic test results, but also allow an exploration of your knowledge of when and how you would use such tests; the indications, appropriateness and limitations of testing; and how test results will influence your clinical management. Example topics to revise and familiarize yourself with are listed below.

Examples of data interpretation topics

Radiological images (indications, anatomy, pathology, further testing, management)
- Ultrasound (identify transabdominal vs transvaginal)
- Hysterosalpinogram
- MRI/CT scanning

Endoscopic images (indications, anatomy, landmarks, pathology, further testing, management, complications)
- Hysteroscopy
- Cystoscopy
- Laparoscopy

General clinical images (identification and management)
- Pathology
- Complications

Examples of data interpretation topics *(continued)*

Pathology specimens/slides/results
- Lower genital tract microscopy (sexually transmitted infections, bacterial vaginosis, candida)
- Vulval disease
- Cervical cytology
- Cervical intraepithelial neoplasia
- Endometrium (functional, inactive, hyperplastic, cancerous)
- Ovarian cysts

Endocrinology/biochemical results
- β-hCG, FSH, LH, prolactin, oestradiol, day 21 progesterone, androgens – ovarian and adrenal (infertility, polycystic ovaries, pregnancy)
- Ovarian tumour markers
- Seminal fluid analysis
- Other – thyroid function, diabetes (GTT, random, HbA1C)

Urological
- Urinanalysis (urinary tract infection, renal disease, pre-eclamspia – 24-hour protein collection, albumin:creatinine ratio, creatinine clearance)
- Urodynamics

Antenatal tests
- Serological screening tests (including haemoglobinopathies, isoimmunization, trisomy and infections)
- Ultrasound, including booking, nuchal screening, anomaly, fetal growth scanning, uterine and umbilical Doppler studies, biophysical profiles
- Immunology results – renal disease/connective tissue disorders and pregnancy
- Pre-eclampsia screen and blood pressure monitoring

Acute obstetrics
- Partogram
- Cardiotocograph
- Fetal blood sample

Acute gynaecology
- Serial β-hCG
- Ultrasound and surgical images (e.g. ectopic, ovarian torsion, trophoblastic disease)

Approach to result interpretation

1. Greet the examiner and be attentive.
2. Listen to and/or read instructions carefully.
3. Maintain a good posture when reading the test result (put your chair in a position that is comfortable for you and sit forward on the front half of the chair with your feet flat on the floor).
4. Handle any source material presented to you by the examiner sparingly and do not move it/fidget excessively (i.e. do not give the impression that this is the first time you have ever seen such a test/image!).
5. Do not answer immediately even if you are certain of the answer. Pause for a few seconds to allow you to compose your thoughts and formulate an answer. This will convey an impression of a sensible and measured clinician.
6. Engage the examiner and ensure eye contact when responding (there is a tendency to stare at the test result and to ignore the examiner).
7. State what the test/image is, then extract the information/describe the key features in a systematic way (avoid criticizing the quality of the image/data provided), identify normal/abnormal results or findings and then give the diagnosis/likely diagnosis supported by your preceding description (e.g. the presence of visible endometriotic peritoneal deposits favours endometriosis as the cause of the filmy tubo-ovarian adhesions, although pelvic inflammatory disease is another possibility). If you do not know the diagnosis then you will still gain some marks for your description.

   Answer the question concisely, but you can expand your answer succinctly if this provides relevant further information demonstrating your understanding (e.g. use of additional, confirmatory tests; suggest what you would normally do presented with these findings).
8. If challenged by the examiner, then reconsider your answer, but if you still believe that your initial interpretation or management plan was a good one, then justify your case with supporting statements in a firm, but courteous manner. If it is clear you have 'messed up', then acknowledge this gracefully and move on to ensure you concentrate fully on the next case/question.
9. The examiner will then ask further questions based upon the test result or provide further tests to be interpreted.
10. Do not worry if the examiner gives you no feedback when moving between cases as, whilst this is unnerving, they will have been instructed not to provide positive or negative reinforcement.
11. Thank the examiner when leaving the station.

Example question and structured mark sheet

OSCE Q – Urodynamics (Data interpretation)

You will be presented with several investigation results. You will be asked to interpret these and answer any supplementary questions that the examiner asks.

Marks will be awarded for:

- Correct interpretation of the results;
- Correct answers to the supplementary questions.

Result A

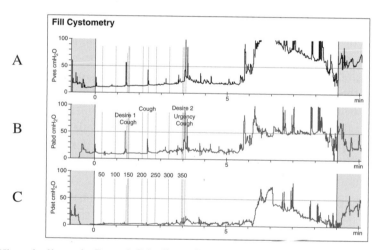

A1. What do lines A, B and C indicate?

A2. What are the indications for performing the above test?

A3. What can cause wandering baselines when there is no real change in the bladder or intra-abdominal pressure?

A4. What is the urodynamic diagnosis in the cystometrogram?

A5. What are the mainstay therapies for the condition?

A6. What are the newer modalities for treating this condition that you are aware of?

A7. What is the significance of a detrusor pressure rise of above 50 cm H_2O?

Result B

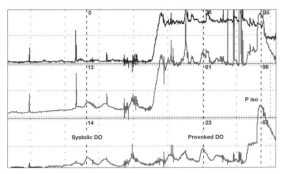

B1. If the patient also leaked with cough in the above cystometrogram, what would your diagnosis be?

B2. What is the significance of voiding studies in this condition?

Result C

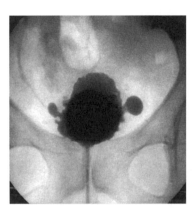

C1. What is the above investigation and what abnormalities can you see?

Structured mark sheet

Result A

A1. What do lines A, B and C indicate? [1]

- A – bladder pressure.
- B – rectal pressure which denotes intra-abdominal pressure.
- C – detrusor pressure.

    0   1

A2. What are the indications for performing the above test? [3]
Multichannel filling and voiding cystometry is recommended in women before surgery for urinary incontinence in the following circumstances:

- Clinical suspicion of detrusor overactivity;
- Previous surgery for stress incontinence or anterior compartment prolapse;
- Symptoms suggestive of voiding dysfunction;
- There is a need to demonstrate the presence of specific abnormalities before undertaking complex reconstructive urological procedures;
- Clinical diagnosis is unclear prior to surgery;
- Initial treatment has failed.

0   1   2   3

A3. What can cause wandering baselines when there is no real change in the bladder or intra-abdominal pressure? [1]
- Rectal drop of the transducer.
- Air bubbles in the catheter.
- Peristaltic wave in the bowel.

0   1

A4. What is the urodynamic diagnosis in the cystometrogram? [1]
Detrusor overactivity – rise in detrusor pressure associated with urgency.

0   1

A5. What are the mainstay therapies for the condition? [1]
Bladder retraining and anticholinergic medications.

0   1

A6. What are the newer modalities for treating this condition that you are aware of? [1]
- Intradetrusor botulinum toxin injection.
- Sacral neuromodulation.

0   1

A7. What is the significance of a detrusor pressure rise of above 50 cm H_2O water? [1]
Need to rule out neurological cause for the detrusor overactivity, e.g. multiple sclerosis.

0   1

Result B

B1. If the patient also leaked with cough in the above cystometrogram, what would your diagnosis be? [2]

Provoked detrusor overactivity as the leak would be associated with detrusor pressure rise. Remember that for urodynamic stress incontinence, the incontinence has to be demonstrable without the detrusor pressure rise.

0   1   2

B2. What is the significance of voiding studies in this condition? [2]

To rule out pre-existing voiding difficulties and as baseline prior to starting anticholinergics, etc, as they can be associated with urinary retention.

0   1   2

Result C

C1. What is the above investigation and what abnormalities can you see? [3]

- Videocystourethrogram taken at videourodynamics.
- Abnormalities seen: trabeculation, diverticuli and vesicoureteric reflux on the right side.

Global score [4]

0   1   2   3   4

Total: /20

Critical appraisal of the medical literature and audit

Almost every OSCE carries a question on critical appraisal of medical literature. The majority of questions are likely to fit into one of five categories:

1. Therapy studies (randomized controlled studies);
2. Diagnostic studies (test accuracy studies);
3. Systematic reviews and meta-analyses;
4. Patient information leaflets;
5. Audits.

It is possible to be presented with other types of studies, e.g. ones on prognosis (cohort study), aetiology (case-control or cohort studies) or efficiency (economic evaluations), but unlikely. However, if the need arises, the principles provided in this chapter can be modified to address all these different types of studies.

Why appraise the medical literature?

Many papers published in medical journals have serious methodological flaws, and most are irrelevant for everyday clinical practice. Although many of you are in the 'user' mode when you look for evidence to support practice, you cannot always find up-to-date and valid pre-appraised summaries and synopses, and it becomes necessary to switch to 'appraiser' mode, roll up your sleeves and try to make sense of the evidence yourself. This process starts with defining the exact clinical question you want answered and finding the relevant paper(s), and only then does appraising them become an issue. However, as you will be given the paper for appraisal in the OSCE, the steps of defining the question, and searching and finding the literature will not be relevant in the exam, and are not covered in this chapter.

So, what does appraisal involve? It involves checking the articles for:

- Validity (methodological soundness);
- Importance (e.g. is a *statistically* significant reduction in BP of 2 mmHg *clinically* significant?);
- Applicability to your patients.

Various checklists exist to help in the appraisal of different types of clinical questions (see www.cebm.net). We cover the important ones in this chapter.

Anatomy of a scientific paper

Most scientific articles have the IMRAD structure – Introduction (or background), Methods (or materials and methods), Results (or findings) and Discussion. They often have an abstract which is also usually structured as IMRAD. All of these sections are important, but some are more important than others. Which are these? This may seem an academic question, but it is not! If you are struggling to make sense of a lengthy article due to time limitation in your OSCE, you will need to prioritize what you read. We recommend that you prioritize the abstract, methods and results. The *abstract* should give you a quick overview of the paper; the *methods* should tell you what was done in the study, from which you can assess its validity; and the *results* should tell you what was found. What about the introduction and the discussion that we know many of you are fond of devoting a lot of time to? If time permits, by all means do read these, but these are secondary to the abstract, methods and results.

General principles in appraising a scientific paper

Step 1: Introduce

Introduce the paper and your purpose: *'I would like to present the appraisal findings of this article by (mention first author) and colleagues, published in (journal name) in (year of publication) on the subject of (subject matter of the paper). I will summarize the appraisal findings, highlighting the study's strengths and weaknesses, and conclude with my interpretation of the findings in terms of implications for clinical practice and for research.'*

Step 2: Define the exact clinical question asked by the paper

The way to define a clinical question is by using the PICOD structure (Table 5.1). You can often get all elements of PICOD from the abstract, although sometimes it is necessary to go through the Methods section to find all the relevant information. Once you have identified your PICOD elements, put these together succinctly in a statement for your examiner. For example: *'This randomized controlled trial evaluates the effectiveness of low-dose aspirin compared to a placebo on the outcomes of pre-eclampsia and perinatal mortality in women at risk of pre-eclampsia.'*

TABLE 5.1 PICOD structure to define a clinical question

Component	Example 1	Example 2
P: Population, Patient or Problem	In women at risk of pre-eclampsia	In pregnant women with swollen legs
I: Intervention (test, treatment or process of care)	Would treatment with low-dose aspirin	Would a Doppler ultrasound be accurate
C: Comparison (placebo, another treatment or the gold standard in a diagnostic accuracy study)	Compared to placebo	Compared to venography as the gold standard
O: Outcome(s)	Lead to reduction in the risk of pre-eclampsia and perinatal mortality?	In diagnosing DVTs?
D: Design of the study	An RCT	A test accuracy study

Step 3: Provide details

Now dive deep into the Methods section, particularly looking at the *inclusion* and *exclusion criteria*. The purpose is to provide more details on PICOD. For example: *'In this study high risk women (population) were defined as women with a previous history of pre-eclampsia, chronic hypertension or diabetes and those who had positive uterine artery Doppler at 12–14 weeks' gestation. The intervention was aspirin at a dose of 75 mg, started at 14 weeks' gestation and continued until 36 weeks. The primary outcomes were pre-eclampsia, defined as … and perinatal death, defined as … The secondary outcomes were ….'*

Step 4: Appraise the study for validity

All the information you need for this will be found in the Methods section. Checklists that will help you with the appraisal of the three common types of articles are provided in the next few pages. It is important to approach your paper with a checklist like these in your mind. Then, your reading of the article will be purposeful and focused as you gather the facts to answer the questions in the checklist. You can then summarize the output from this exercise. For example: *'This is a randomized, allocation-concealed, placebo-controlled, double-blind study. Randomization was achieved with the use of a computer-generated random number list; allocation concealment was accomplished by placing the treatment allocation in opaque envelopes; both the clinician providing the care and the patient were blinded, making the study double-blind. The analysis was by intention-to-treat and the follow-up rate was excellent, with data being available on over 95% of those who were randomized. Thus the methods of this trial are excellent'.*

Of course, if there are any weaknesses in the Methods, you will highlight these also. This step is the backbone of your appraisal. Do a good job with it and do not rush it!

Step 5: Provide the findings

You will find all that you need to address this step in the Results section and the tables and figures of the article. 'Table 1' in most articles is where researchers summarize data on demographic and baseline characteristics of the populations being compared – start with this. Then move on to providing the study findings. Provide confidence intervals around the findings where these are provided. For example: *'The baseline characteristics between the aspirin and placebo group were similar. The main findings were that there was a reduction in pre-eclampsia risk, with a relative risk (RR) of 0.6 and a 95% confidence interval (CI) from 0.5 to 0.8. The study also found that ...'.*

Step 6: Put the study findings in the context of the existing evidence

A judgement can almost never be made about the value of an intervention or test based on one paper alone – you need to weigh up the balance of evidence. For this step, you may find the Discussion section of the article helpful, if the authors have taken the trouble to place their study in the context of existing evidence. Unfortunately, the Discussion section of articles is generally abused by authors: they shamelessly fill it with irrelevant curiosities that they were unable to place elsewhere, and often put spin on their findings. So, skim through the Discussion, but if you find that the authors have written about previous studies on this subject, stop and take this in. Hopefully, using the information in the Discussion and your pre-existing knowledge, you can put the study in context. If you cannot, you may have to state to the examiner that you would want to find out more about what other studies on this subject show before you could decide on whether the evidence should be incorporated into clinical practice. Your efforts should produce something of this sort: *'The findings from the study are consistent with over 40 other studies summarized in a Cochrane review'.*

Step 7: Make your recommendation for practice and research

There is no point in appraising a paper unless you come to some judgement about whether it is appropriate for guiding clinical practice or further research. Steps 4, 5 and 6 above will contribute to your judgement: *'As this is a high quality study that shows substantial reduction in pre-eclampsia and perinatal death, and the findings are consistent with other studies on this subject, I will recommend aspirin therapy to women at risk of pre-eclampsia* [clinical implication]. *Further research may be required to examine the role of aspirin in other high risk groups such as those with renal disease* [research implication]'.

Appraising a therapy paper (randomized controlled trials)

Checklist to appraise a therapy article

1. Are the results valid?

- Is the assignment of patients randomized? (*appropriate methods are: random number tables and computer generated random numbers*)
- Is the allocation of patient concealed? [*appropriate methods are: opaque envelopes, third party randomization, distant (telephone or Internet) allocation*]
- Are patients, health workers and study personnel 'blind' to treatment?
- Are patients analyzed in the groups to which they were randomized? (*'intention to treat' analysis*)
- Are all patients who entered the trial properly accounted for and attributed at its conclusion?
- Is follow-up complete?
- Are the groups similar at the start of the trial? (*normally presented in 'Table 1' of the article*)
- Aside from the experimental intervention, are the groups treated equally?

Checklist to appraise a therapy article *(continued)*

- Was the study adequately powered?*
- Was ethical approval obtained for the study?*

2. What are the results (i.e. their importance)?

- How large is the treatment effect? [*reported as relative risks, odds ratios, absolute risks or numbers needed to treat (NNT)*]
- How precise is the treatment effect? (*95% confidence interval*)

3. Will the results help me in caring for my patients (applicability)?

- Can the results be applied to my patients?
- Are all clinically important outcomes considered?
- What are the likely benefits? Are they worth the potential harms and costs?

*These items do not strictly relate to 'validity'; nevertheless, they are important and should be part of the appraisal process.

Appraising a diagnosis article

Checklist to appraise a diagnosis article

1. Are the results valid?

- Does the patient sample include an appropriate spectrum of patients to whom the test will be applied in clinical practice?
- Were the test and reference (gold) standard results obtained by assessors blinded to each other?
- Did everyone get *both* the test and the reference standard?
- Is the test described fully?
- Is the reference standard described fully?

2. What are the results?

- What are the results? (*sensitivity, specificity, predictive values or likelihood ratios*)
- What is their precision? (*95% confidence intervals*)

3. Will the results help me in caring for my patients?

- Are the results applicable to my patients?
- Will the results change my management?
- Will patients be better off as a result of the test?

Appraising a systematic review or meta-analysis

Checklist to appraise a systematic review or meta-analysis

1. Are the results valid?
- Does the article address a clearly focused question? (*i.e. are the PICOD elements clearly defined?*)
- Are the criteria used to select articles for inclusion appropriate?
- Is the literature search comprehensive? (*MEDLINE, EMBASE, Cochrane Library, CINRHL, searches for abstracts, hand-searching etc*)
- Is the validity of the included studies appraised? (*using checklists like those given above*)
- Did two or more reviewers extract the data independently?
- Are the results consistent from study to study?
- Is there an assessment for publication bias? (*e.g. funnel plot analysis*)

2. What are the results?
- What are the results of the study?
- How precise are the results? (*95% confidence intervals*)

3. Will the results help me in caring for my patients?
- Can the results be applied to my patient care?
- Are all clinically relevant outcomes considered?
- Are the benefits worth the harms and costs?

Appraising a patient information leaflet

A patient information leaflet can be appraised under the broad headings of validity, clarity, credibility, currency and format.

At the end of the assessment, do not forget to provide an overall judgement on the quality of the information leaflet. For example, you may state: '*In summary, this information leaflet has many strengths* [name a few] *and a few minor weaknesses* [name a few], *and thus with minor modifications, I would be happy to use it with the patients that I look after*'.

Checklist to appraise an information leaflet

- Is the aim clearly stated?
- **Validity:**
  - Is the information accurate and comprehensive?
  - Are the sources of information given? (*e.g. patient information leaflet may have been based on a guideline, literature review or a consensus process*)
- **Clarity** and presentation:
  - Is the language simple and non-medical?
  - Are there annotated diagrams?
  - Have boxes and bullet points been used?
  - Have the authors used a question and answer format?
  - Have they provided useful summaries? (*ideally at the beginning and at the end*)
  - Has there been good use of colour?
- **Credibility:**
  - Is authorship of the patient information leaflet given? (*it is not good enough to state, 'This patient information leaflet was produced by 'x' or 'y' society' – the actual authors' names should be provided*)
  - Is there a 'conflict of interest' declaration stated by any authors? (*this is particularly important for any patient information leaflet that carries recommendations for commercial products, including specific drugs*)
- **Currency:**
  - Is there a creation date?
  - Is there an expiry or revision date?
- **Format:** Can the leaflet be folded to fit into a handbag? (*it needs to be A5 size or smaller*)
- Is there a section on 'Further information and help'?

Appraising an audit

If you understand the six steps of an audit, then designing or appraising an audit becomes an easy task. The six steps are detailed below, using an audit of colposcopy referrals from primary care to secondary care as an example where appropriate.

Step 1: Define criteria and standards

Many people are confused by the difference between the terms criterion and standard. The difference is best illustrated with an example. A 'criterion' for a colposcopy referral audit may be: 'women with moderate dyskaryosis should be referred after 1 abnormal smear'. A 'standard' related to that criterion may be: 'At least 90% of women with a moderate dyskaryosis should be seen within 4 weeks of referral'.

Criteria and standards often come from national or professional body guidelines (e.g. the RCOG Green Top Guidelines often provide 'auditable standards'), policy statements, reviews of practice (i.e. previous audits or surveys) or consensus by stakeholders.

Step 2: Measure current practice

- Decide whether this needs to be:
  - **Prospective** (time consuming, but provides more complete data; however, this approach may suffer from the Hawthorne effect of improvement in practice while the audit is being conducted); or
  - **Retrospective** (quicker to do, but there may be a great deal of missing data).
- Consider the **sampling** frame – all in a defined period, random, or arbitrary?
- Consider the **sample size** (balance between precision and feasibility). (People often discuss 'power calculation'. This is an irrelevant phrase in the context of audits, as audits are not designed to test hypothesis, and consideration of type I and type II errors and power do not apply to audits.)
- **Design (and pilot) the data collection form/pro-forma** (make it as simple as possible – just collecting the essential data for the audit; not looking for 'interesting facts' and burdening the data collectors).
- Decide on **data entry** into a database (e.g. Excel).

Step 3: Analyze data

- **Consider possibility of sampling/selection bias.**
- **Quantitative analysis** (e.g. what proportion of women with moderate dyskaryosis were referred to the colposcopy unit?).
- **Qualitative analysis** (why were some missed?).
- Decide on the format of presentation of data (e.g. pie charts, bar charts, proportions).

Step 4: Present results

- Anticipate reactions.
- Do this sensitively; do not assign personal blame ('hard on issues; soft on individuals').
- Use various methods, e.g.:
  - Audit meetings;
  - Hospital e-mails;
  - Letters;
  - 'Quality improvement journals' (if your audit has a wider relevance outside your own setting).

Step 5: Identify (as well as disseminate and implement) strategies to improve the care

- Involve all stakeholders.
- Consider revising guidelines.
- Consider multifaceted approaches.
- Consider resource implications.

Step 6: Close the audit loop

Plan a re-audit at an appropriate time to check the changes have been made (process audit) and outcomes are improved (outcome audit).

Example question and structured mark sheet

OSCE Q – A randomized trial (Critical appraisal)

Candidate's instructions

This is a preparatory station. Read and appraise the article titled 'Usefulness of aspirin therapy in high-risk pregnant women with abnormal uterine artery Doppler ultrasound at 14–16 weeks' pregnancy: Randomized controlled clinical trial' by Ebrashy et al, published in the *Croatian Medical Journal*.

You may make notes on this article, and take the notes with you to the next station, where you will discuss its value and limitations with the examiner.

(Note: The article will of course be given to you in the exam, but to reproduce it here would be an infringement of copyright regulations. Please therefore download a free copy of this article from the journal website at:

www.cmj.hr/2005/46/5/16158479.pdf; alternatively you can ask your librarian to obtain this article for you.)

Marks will be awarded for:

Critically appraising the article for its merits and weaknesses.

Examiner's instructions

This is a critical appraisal station. At this station, the candidate has 14 minutes to discuss the strengths and weaknesses of the article titled, 'Usefulness of aspirin therapy in high-risk pregnant women with abnormal uterine artery Doppler ultrasound at 14–16 weeks' pregnancy: Randomized controlled clinical trial' by Ebrashy et al, published in the *Croatian Medical Journal*. You can prompt the candidate if necessary, but this requirement should be reflected in the marks awarded.

Structured mark sheet

Information about the study [3]
- Details of the article (author, year, journal): Ebrashy et al, 2005, *CMJ*
- Details of the study (**PICOD**):
  - **P**opulation: Women at high risk of PET due to abnormal uterine artery Doppler at 14–16 weeks;
  - **I**ntervention: Aspirin 75 mg daily;
    Comparison: No treatment;
  - **O**utcome(s): Pre-eclampsia, growth restriction, preterm birth, mode of delivery, neonatal outcomes;
  - **D**esign: RCT.
- Objectives clear? Yes.

0   1   2   3

Validity (methods) [5]
- Appropriately randomized? Yes, computer-generated random numbers.
- Appropriately concealed? Yes, with opaque envelopes.
- Blinded? No.
- Intention-to-treat (ITT) analysis? Yes.

- Good follow-up rates? Yes (3/139 = 2% were lost to follow-up).
- Adequate power to answer the primary research question? Yes.
- Was ethical approval obtained? Yes.

0   1   2   3   4   5

Results [4]

- *Primary outcomes* (relative risks, odds ratios, mean differences): Pre-eclampsia developed in 35% of women receiving aspirin and 62% of women in the control group (P = 0.003), with severe pre-eclampsia developing in 8% and 23% of women (P = 0.215), respectively.
- *Secondary outcomes*: In the group of women receiving aspirin, 19% of newborns suffered from IUGR as opposed to 32% of newborns in the control group (P = 0.106). There was no significant difference between the two groups in the rate of preterm delivery (P = 0.080), mode of delivery (P = 0.971), Apgar score < 5 after 1 minute (P = 0.273) and after 5 minutes (P = 0.941), maternal or neonatal bleeding (P = 0.948) and neonatal birth weight (P = 0.399).

0   1   2   3   4

Discussion [4]

- Strengths and weaknesses of the study. Summarize your appraisal above.
- Put the study in the context of other evidence. Look at the discussion of the article to help you with this.
- Implications for practice (and *your* view on this!).
- Implications for research (and *your* view on this!).

0   1   2   3   4

Global score [4]

0   1   2   3   4

Total: /20

| 6 | **Equipment, surgery and practical procedures** |

This chapter addresses common surgical interventions in O&G relevant to the MRCOG Part 2 examination. When asked to discuss patient management in relation to surgical intervention you should consider relevant pre-, peri- and post-operative factors. This chapter summarizes key issues in terms of preoperative work up, description and use of surgical equipment, generic operative technique and approach for specific procedures, and how to prevent and recognize complications.

Preoperative assessment and consent

Preoperative assessment

Once a surgical intervention has been decided upon, thought must turn to the preoperative preparation of patients in order to minimize complications. Hospital admission should be kept to a minimum both for the convenience of patients and to reduce risk of hospital acquired infections [e.g. methicillin-resistant *Staphylococcus aureus* (MRSA)] and venous thromboembolism (VTE). In addition, consider:

- General advice where relevant (e.g. stop smoking, reduce weight).
- Prophylaxis against infection and VTE (see below).
- Physical status. A five-category preoperative classification system from the American Society of Anesthesiologists (ASA) has been widely adopted:

  I   Healthy patient
  II   Mild systemic disease (no functional limitations)
  III Severe systemic disease (definite functional limitations)

IV   Severe systemic disease that is a constant threat to life
V   Moribund patient who is not expected to survive without the operation

- Preoperative investigation will be dictated by the type of procedure (elective vs emergency; major vs minor operation) and the ASA classification of physical status. Most procedures in O&G require only a full blood count (FBC) and a blood group and save depending upon the risk of bleeding and preoperative haemoglobin level.

Preoperative investigations

- *Full blood count* (abnormal uterine bleeding, > 60-years-old, risk of bleeding during operation, point-of-care testing in operating theatre unavailable)
- *Blood group and save* (significant risk of bleeding/requiring blood transfusion – consider cross-match if risk of bleeding high, preoperative anaemia or rapid cross-matching unavailable)
- *Coagulation screen* (e.g. taking warfarin, on renal dialysis, liver or vascular disease)
- Blood gases (cardiorespiratory disease)
- *Sickle cell test* (ethnicity with higher risk of sickle cell disease or trait)
- *Renal function tests* (> 60-years-old, diabetes, hypertension, on medications that affect renal function, known renal disease)

Consent

In any discussion pertaining to surgical interventions, the concept of consent cannot be ignored. Candidates must understand the importance legally and ethically of obtaining valid consent prior to medical intervention. The issues around consent have been well documented and are beyond the scope of this revision book. Here we highlight three key principles:

1. If consent is to be considered valid it must be given voluntarily by an appropriately informed person who has the capacity to consent to the intervention.
2. The clinician providing the treatment or investigation is responsible for ensuring that the patient has given valid consent before treatment.
3. Obtaining consent may be delegated to another suitably trained and qualified health professional as long as they have sufficient knowledge and understanding of the proposed intervention, including the risks involved, so as to provide any information the patient may require.

The RCOG has developed some procedure-specific advice for clinicians, outlining the risks and side effects of common O&G procedures, which should be useful to the prospective MRCOG Part 2 candidate (available at www.rcog.org.uk/index.asp?PageID=686).

Fundamental principles of surgery

Patient positioning

Most operative procedures in O&G involve positioning patients to ensure good access to the pelvis and perineum.

- **Trendelenburg position:** supine position with the feet higher than the head (e.g. abdominal hysterectomy).
- **Lithotomy position:** supine position with hips/knees flexed and abducted (e.g. hysteroscopy, vaginal surgery, instrumental delivery).
- **Lloyd–Davis position:** lithotomy position with reduced flexion of the hips (e.g. laparoscopic surgery).

Surgical incisions

Laparotomy in O&G practice uses the following two incisions:

- **Lower transverse** (Pfannensteil = curved; Maylard = curved + rectus muscles cut; Cohen = straight + blunt entry);
- **Vertical** (midline; paramedian).

Compared with a vertical incision, transverse incisions limit exploration of the upper abdomen, are associated with greater blood loss, are more prone to haematoma formation and result in greater paraesthesia of the overlying skin. However, transverse approaches give better cosmetic results, less postoperative pain and are associated with a lower incidence of wound dehiscence and hernia formation.

Be prepared to discuss the rationale, advantages and disadvantages of each type of incision, and when you would use them. Remember, you will never be criticized for performing a midline entry, especially where access is likely to be limited (e.g. the obese patient, adhesions are expected – previous surgery, infection, endometriosis).

Rationale for abdominal incisions

- Abdominal incisions are based on anatomical principles
- They must allow adequate assess to the abdomen
- They should be capable of being extended if required
- Ideally, muscle fibres should be split rather than cut
- Nerves should not be divided

Suture selection

A suture is any strand of material used to approximate tissue or ligate vessels. The material used should provide uniform tensile strength throughout healing and knot security, induce little tissue reaction (scarring), be resistant to infection, have a favourable absorption profile and be non-allergenic. Sutures are either *absorbable*, providing temporary wound support until the wound heals well enough to withstand normal stress (broken down by enzymatic action or hydrolysis), or *non-absorbable* (Table 6.1).

TABLE 6.1   Types of suture commonly used in obstetric and gynaecological surgery

Absorbable	Non-absorbable
Surgical gut	Stainless steel (clips)
Polyglactin (Vicryl)	Silk
Polyglycolic acid (Dexon)	Nylon (Dermalon)
Poliglecaprone (Monocryl)	Polypropylene (Prolene)
Polydioxanone (PDS)	Braided synthetics (Dacron)

Sutures are no longer needed when a wound has reached maximum strength. Thus, in general, consider non-absorbable sutures or delayed absorbable sutures for slowly healing tissues (e.g. skin, fascia) and absorbable sutures for rapidly healing tissues (mucous membranes, e.g. peritoneum).

Be prepared to discuss when to use particular types of suture and needle (cutting vs blunt needle point; absorbable vs non-absorbable; monofilament vs multifilament; suture size; patient characteristics, tissues being approximated; when to remove skin sutures).

Electrosurgery

In view of the widespread use of electrosurgery in gynaecological practice, the aspiring MRCOG II candidate should be able to display an understanding of the fundamental principles and applications of this energy modality. Key points to understand are:

- **Electrical generators**. These convert mains AC electric current (50 Hz) to high frequency current (200 kHz–3.3 MHz), avoiding muscle contraction and electrocution.

- **Electrical waveforms**. Electrosurgical generators can produce a variety of electrical waveforms. A constant waveform produces a rapid and intense temperature rise (> 100° C), which vaporizes and easily cuts through tissue (pure cut). If the duty cycle generated is interrupted (an intermittent or modulated waveform), less heat is produced, resulting in different tissue effects ('blended cut'). As the duty cycle is progressively reduced, cutting (vaporization) properties wane and desiccation (coagulation providing haemostasis) becomes the dominant tissue effect (80–100° C).

- **Heat and tissue effects**. These are produced whenever current flows through tissues and are dependent upon the resistance of the tissues and the density of current flow. Eschar deposited upon electrodes or charring of tissues increases resistance to current flow, whereas the use of a fine electrode, end on, with 'sparking' in close proximity to, rather than direct contact with, tissue and longer activation times maximizes current density and heat production. The 'cutting' waveform can be used to coagulate and the 'coagulation' waveform can be used to cut, depending upon how the electrode is used.

- **Monopolar vs bipolar circuits**. In bipolar electrosurgery, both the active and return electrode functions occur at the site of surgery, whereas with monopolar diathermy, the current flows through the patient to a more distant return electrode. Bipolar circuits are inherently safer because the current path is confined to the intervening tissue, reducing the risk of stray current and alternate site burns.

- **Safety**. Modern electrosurgical generators have greatly reduced the risks of current diversion and unintended burns. The operator must adopt good practice (e.g. store electrodes in insulated holders, activate electrodes only under direct vision in close or direct proximity to tissues, use the lowest available effective power setting and, ideally, bipolar circuits). Laparoscopic surgery requires a higher level of vigilance to avoid the additional risks of direct coupling (inadvertent contact between the activated electrode and another conducting instrument) and capacitive coupling (use of mixed plastic/metal cannulate preventing dissipation of capacitively coupled electrical energy).

Miscellaneous

Be prepared to discuss other general points relating to surgery, e.g. the need for catheterization; when to leave drains; types of drain; purpose of postoperative review; duration of stay; discharge and follow-up.

Preventing complications

Anticipate potential problems and arrange adequate time for surgery, help from anaesthetists/urologists/general surgeons, bowel preparation. Common factors associated with an increased risk of surgical complications include:

- Risks of surgery vs benefits (remember the Hippocratic Oath);
- Obesity;
- Adhesions (previous surgery, infection, endometriosis);
- Pelvic cancer;
- Radical surgery.

Infection

Surgical site and hospital-acquired infections are 'hot topics' and so, in any discussion of operative interventions, an appreciation of the risk of infection and both primary and secondary prevention is important. In O&G practice the most likely pathogens to be encountered are Gram-negative bacilli, enterococci, Group B streptococci and anaerobes.

Prevention of infection begins preoperatively by identifying those patient groups at increased risk (diabetics, obese, smokers, steroid use, malnourished, acute admissions) and screening where necessary (see below). Perioperative measures used to reduce infection risk include:

- Use of appropriate antibiotics (up to 1 hour prior to skin incision) to reduce the microbial burden of intraoperative contamination to a level that cannot overwhelm host defences;
- Restricted use of surgical shaves;
- Use of antiseptic agents for preoperative skin preparation at the incision site (e.g. iodophors, alcohol-containing products and chlorhexidine gluconate);
- Careful surgical technique (minimize tissue trauma).

Information relating to two serious and topical postoperative infections, namely methicillin-resistant *Staphylococcus aureus* (MRSA) and *Clostridium difficile*, is presented below.

Methicillin-resistant *Staphylococcus aureus* (MRSA)

Staphylococcus aureus, including MRSA, is found in human skin, particularly in the anterior nares (nose – up to 30% of the population are nasal carriers), axilla (armpit) and perineum (groin). Clinical infection with MRSA occurs either from the patient's own resident MRSA (asymptomatic carrier) or by cross-infection from another person [healthcare worker or visitor (asymptomatic carrier)] or directly/indirectly from a clinically infected patient.

- **Prevention:**
  - Screening;
  - Hand hygiene (antiseptics, use alcohol-based hand rubs between patients);
  - Regularly clean environment;
  - Dress skin wounds;
  - Isolate infected patients;
- **Screening.** The transmission of MRSA and the risk of MRSA infection can only be addressed effectively if measures are taken to identify MRSA carriers as potential sources and treat them to reduce the risk of transmission. This requires screening of patient populations for MRSA carriage either before or on admission to identify carriers and implement a decolonization regimen. However, local practice to reduce the risk of MRSA infection (level of screening and decontamination regimens) varies in the absence of consistent, evidence-based advice. Some adopt selective screening of higher risk groups (previously known to be MRSA positive; orthopaedic/cardiothoracic/neurosurgical patients; immunocompromised; admission from nursing homes; emergency admissions) and others employ universal screening.
- **Screening samples.** Anterior nares (nose) – the most common carriage site for MRSA, and most patients positive at other sites have positive results from nose samples (but a small proportion do not). The secondary sites to sample are the axilla and perineum.
- **Decolonization.** This comprises the use of an antibacterial shampoo and body wash daily (e.g. Aquasept), and the application of an antibacterial nasal cream (e.g. mupirocin nasal ointment) three times a day for five days with the aim of eradicating the organism. The purpose of decolonisation is to reduce the risk of both the patient developing an MRSA infection with their own MRSA during medical or surgical treatment and transmission of MRSA to another patient.
- **Treatment of clinical MRSA infection:**
  - Isolation (side rooms) to reduce the risk of transmission to other patients;
  - Decolonization regimen;
  - Antibiotics, e.g. vancomycin and teicoplanin.

Clostridium difficile

This is a spore-forming, Gram-positive bacillus carried in the gastrointestinal tract of a small proportion of adults in the community, with higher rates in hospital patients. Antibiotic-associated colitis caused by *Clostridium difficile* exhibits a spectrum of disease, from diarrhoea through colitis to toxic megacolon and pseudomembranous colitis, which can be fatal.

- **Primary prevention:**
  - Restricted use of antibiotics;
  - Routine infection control procedures (particularly hand washing by healthcare staff);
  - Patient education and hand washing;
  - Environmental cleaning, in particular of toilet areas.
- **Secondary prevention**. Infection control procedures should be strictly adhered to during an outbreak to prevent cross-infection:
  - Isolation in a room with en-suite toilet facilities;
  - Hand decontamination for both staff and patients;
  - Use of disposable gloves and plastic aprons for the care of patients with diarrhoea;
  - Daily cleaning to reduce spore load in the environment, particularly linen and patient equipment;
  - Restrict admissions to the unit.
- **Management**. Withdrawal of antibiotics and rehydration will resolve most cases. Although antibiotics precipitate the disease, antibiotic therapy with metronidazole and/or vancomycin can be used to resolve it.

Venous thromboembolism

Pelvic surgery is a major risk for venous thromboembolism (VTE). Do not forget to consider prophylaxis against VTE when discussing operative procedures in O&G.

For *gynaecological surgery*, the National Institute for Clinical Excellence (NICE) recommends:

- Mechanical prophylaxis using graduated elastic compression stockings and/or intermittent pneumatic compression devices, in the absence of patient-related risk factors.
- Mechanical prophylaxis plus low molecular weight heparin (LMWH) if there are any patient-related risk factors [e.g. age > 60 years, obesity (body mass index $\geq$ 30 kg/m^2), personal/family history of VTE, inherited thrombophilias, pregnancy or puerperium, use of oral contraceptives or HRT].

> **Other measures to avoid VTE associated with gynaecological surgery**
>
> - Early mobilization
> - Avoid dehydration
> - Advise patients to consider stopping combined oral contraceptives 4 weeks before elective surgery
> - Inform patients that immobility associated with continuous travel of > 3 hours in the 4 weeks before or after surgery may increase the risk of VTE
> - Encourage patients to wear stockings from admission until they return to their usual levels of mobility

Women having a *caesarean section* are at increased risk of VTE. The choice of method of prophylaxis should take into account the risk of VTE (e.g. increased risk with emergency caesarean sections, age > 35 years, obesity, medical complications). Although practice varies between obstetric units in the UK, current data show that the majority of women undergoing caesarean section (elective or emergency) procedures have LMWH.

Management of common surgical complications in O&G

- **Bladder injury**. Repair in two layers with absorbable sutures + continuous bladder drainage by a suprapubic or transurethral catheter, maintained on free flow for 7–10 days.
- **Ureteric injury**. Call urologist; stent lumen or, if transected, end-to-end anastomosis (> 6 cm from insertion into bladder) vs reimplantation into bladder (< 6 cm from insertion into bladder).
- **Bowel injury**. Isolate with swabs to avoid leakage of bowel contents; call bowel surgeon; repair with fine (e.g. 3/0) absorbable sutures or bowel resection and anastomosis.
- **Vascular injury**. Call vascular surgeon: laparotomy (if laparoscopic injury); direct compression to control blood loss; use of atraumatic vascular clamps to occlude the injured vessel, avoiding intimal crush injury, blood/volume replacement; expose injury site; repair vessel wall with precise (intima-to-intima apposition); consider grafting depending upon extent of injury.

Endoscopic surgery

Endoscopic procedures

The three most common endoscopic techniques in gynaecology are:

1. **Hysteroscopy** – direct visualization of the uterine cavity;
2. **Cystoscopy** – direct visualization of the bladder;
3. **Laparoscopy** – direct visualization of the peritoneal cavity.

Hysteroscopy

- **Technique**:
  - Remove air bubbles;
  - Insertion with minimal distension pressure to optimize view;
  - Systematic inspection of uterine cavity (both tubal ostia, fundus, anterior/posterior/side walls, isthmus, panoramic view of cavity and cervical canal).
- **Diagnostic indications**:
  - Abnormal uterine bleeding;
  - Infertility;
  - Recurrent pregnancy loss;
  - Abnormal glandular cervical smears.
- **Common pathologies**: endometrial hyperplasia and cancer; polyps; fibroids; adhesions; congenital uterine anomalies.
- **Operative**: biopsy; polypectomy; myomectomy; uteroplasty; ablation/resection of endometrium; sterilization; removal of foreign bodies within the genital tract.

Cystoscopy

- **Technique**:
  - Remove air bubbles;
  - Inspection of urethra and insertion into urethra/bladder;
  - Systematic inspection of bladder [neck, trigone, ureteric orifices interureteric ridge, bladder floor, side walls, bladder dome (air bubble)].
- **Diagnostic indications**:
  - Urinary symptoms (urgency–frequency syndrome, painful bladder syndrome);
  - Suspected operative trauma;
  - Suspected anatomical lesions;

- Haematuria;
- Staging for gynaecological malignancy.
- **Common pathologies**: interstitial cystitis; diverticuli; calculi; foreign bodies; carcinoma.
- **Operative**: biopsy; cannulation of ureters to assist laparoscopic surgery; ensure correct positioning of urethral tapes (e.g. TVT); insertion of suprapubic catheter under direct vision; bladder neck injection (bulking agent); botulinum toxin.

Laparoscopy

- **Technique**:
  - Dorso-lithotomy positioning of the patient (Trendelenburg; Lloyd–Davis);
  - 'Bottom end' – disinfect vagina, empty the urinary bladder, insert uterine manipulator (if applicable);
  - Establish pneumoperitoneum (insert the Veress needle through a vertical, 1-cm intraumbilical incision; prior to insertion, the spring mechanism is checked on the needle to help avoid visceral puncture, and insufflator flow/pressure is checked)
  - Check intraperitoneal placement (drop test; high flow; low pressure);
  - Obtain sufficient pneumoperitoneum (25 mmHg);
  - Insert 10–12 mm umbilical trocar through the Veress needle incision (vertically with slight pelvic tilt);
  - Confirm entry into the peritoneal cavity (visualization), lower the intra-abdominal pressure (15 mmHg), Trendelenburg position;
  - Systematic inspection of pelvis (uterus, adnexae, utero-vesical pouch, pouch of Douglas, uterosacral ligaments, peritoneal sidewalls, ovarian fossae, upper abdomen).
- **Diagnostic indications**:
  - Infertility (adhesions – evidence of prior pelvic infection, congenital and acquired structural abnormalities of the uterus, endometriosis, Fallopian tube patency, feasibility of tubal reconstructive surgery);
  - Acute pelvic pain (acute pelvic inflammatory disease (PID), endometriosis, adnexal pathology/cystic accidents (haemorrhage, rupture, torsion), ectopic pregnancy);
  - Appendicitis;
  - Chronic pelvic pain (adhesions, endometriosis, chronic PID, adnexal pathology/cysts).
- **Common pathologies**: endometriosis; adhesions; pelvic infection; adnexal pathology (tubo-ovarian cysts, abscesses, masses, torsion, ectopic gestations).

- **Operative**: biopsy; tubal sterilization; resection/ablation of endometriosis, ovarian cystectomy/oophorectomy; salpingectomy; myomectomy; hysterectomy.

Example descriptions of surgical instruments: key features of endoscopic equipment

Hysteroscopes
- Telescope (rigid or flexible) and diameter
- Proximal eye piece
- Angle of distal lens – usually 0°, 25°, 30° (look at the tip to see whether the lens is offset or look along the barrel of the scope as the distal lens angle is often inscribed along with the surgical manufacturer's name and diameter of instrument)
- Light source attachment
- Inflow port + Luer's lock (single channel, diagnostic set up)
- Inflow and outflow (continuous flow, operative set up) ports
- Operative working channel

Cystoscopes
- Telescope (rigid or flexible) and diameter
- Angle of distal lens – usually 0°, 12°, 30°, 70°, 120°
- Outer sheath and diameter
- Obturator
- Bridge (locking mechanism to hold telescope within the sheath)
- Light source attachment
- Working channel (often two for ureteric cannulation)

Laparoscopes
- Telescope and diameter
- Angle of distal lens – usually 0° or 30°
- Light source attachment
- Ancillary instrumentation (including trocars, traumatic and atraumatic graspers, scissors, energy modalities – monopolar diathermy, bipolar diathermy, ultrasonic instruments, advanced electrosurgical instrumentation)

Describing endoscopic instrumentation

Basic endoscopic examination requires the following equipment:

- Endoscope (rod lens or fibre-optic) for direct visualization within body cavity or hollow viscus;
- High intensity light source and cable to provide illumination;
- Camera with coupling lens and cable to video monitor to transmit and magnify image;
- Distension media (conductive or non-conductive) to distend a body cavity or hollow viscus;
- Ancillary instruments to manipulate, biopsy and operate.

Surgical instruments and interventions

You may be asked about common operative procedures in O&G and the instrumentation used in them. To aid revision we have provided summaries of the instruments and interventions you should be familiar with.

Surgical instruments

If asked to describe and/or assemble surgical instruments, then concentrate on the following key points:

- When presented with an instrument, handle it in a steady, systematic fashion and hold it/assemble it in the way it is intended to be used. When you are nervous there is a tendency to manipulate the instrument excessively and this can give the impression that you lack familiarity with the equipment, so handle it in a purposeful but sparing fashion.
- Do not answer the examiner's questions immediately even if you are certain of the answer. Pause for a few seconds before answering to allow you to compose your thoughts and formulate an answer.
- You can state what the equipment is and then proceed to describe its key features, or begin with the description and then state what it is and what you would use it for.

Instruments you should be prepared to describe

Gynaecology
- Basic surgical instruments, retractors and sutures
- Endoscopes + ancillary equipment

Obstetrics
- Basic surgical instruments, retractors and sutures
- Forceps and vacuum devices
- Fetal blood sampling equipment
- Tamponade balloons

Top tip!

Ask a scrub nurse/senior colleague to talk you through various pieces of equipment – names, key features, assembly and uses.

General surgical instruments used in O&G

Dissecting forceps (toothed and non-toothed)
Use: To handle tissue during dissection and suturing
Examples: Bonney, McIndoe, Gillies, DeBakey

Tissue forceps
Use: To handle tissue during dissection
Examples: Lanes, Littlewood, Allis, Green-Armitage, Babcock, Duval

Haemostatic 'artery' forceps
Use: To provide haemostasis by occluding bleeding points or small vascular pedicle
Examples: Mosquito, Spencer Wells, Kocher, Lahey

Hysterectomy clamps
Use: To secure vascular tissue pedicles at hysterectomy prior to mobilizing and tying
Examples: Bonney, Heaney, Zeppelin, Moynihan, Lahey cholecystectomy

---

General surgical instruments used in O&G *(continued)*

Abdominal hand held retractors
Use: To expose the operating field
Examples: Langenbeck, Czerny, Morris, Doyen, Deaver, De Lee

Topics to prepare for discussion: instruments, design and function.

Obstetric procedures

Repair of episiotomy and tears

The objective is to provide haemostasis and approximate disrupted tissue to aid healing (do not apply excessive tension as this will induce ischaemia, pain and poor healing).

1. Adequate light and exposure, systematic inspection, regional or local anaesthesia (e.g. 1% lidocaine).
2. Appropriate suture material (Cochrane review recommends synthetic suture materials, e.g. polyglycolic acid, or polyglactin, e.g. vicryl rapide® 2/0).
3. Leave small, non-bleeding lacerations to heal naturally by secondary intention.
4. Identify apex of tear, apply continuous locking or non-locking suture to appose edges of vaginal mucosa symmetrically without excessive tension (use anatomic landmarks to guide, e.g. hymenal ring, pigmentation of perineum).
5. Once the posterior vaginal fourchette is reached, the needle is passed through the mucosa to be brought out into the subcutaneous tissue of the perineal body, the first encountered perineal muscles approximated and the suture tied with the knot buried.
6. Use interrupted sutures to close remainder of torn muscles/tissues.
7. Close the perineal skin, starting at the distal apex with a continuous, subcutaneous suture and bury the knot at the proximal end.
8. Check for haemostasis, check adequacy of vaginal introitus with digital examination and perform gentle rectal examination with consent ± 100 mg diclofenac/1 g paracetamol suppository.

Alternative techniques include separate, continuous closure of deep and superficial perineal muscles; using the same continuous suture to close the skin.

Repair of third-/fourth-degree tears

1. Perform in theatre with a regional anaesthetic (ensure adequate light, exposure, assistance and instruments).
2. Retrieve retracted torn ends of the external anal sphincter and approximate either end-to-end or using the overlap technique using a monofilament suture material [e.g. polydioxanone (PDS®)].
3. Use intraoperative and postoperative broad-spectrum antibiotics (e.g. co-amoxiclav/cephalexin + metronidazole) and laxatives [e.g. lactulose and ispaghula husk (Fybogel)] and arrange follow-up (preferably in a specialist perineal trauma clinic).

Topics to prepare for discussion: indications for episiotomy; definition of tears; causation; long-term complications; mode of subsequent delivery if third-/fourth-degree tear.

Fetal blood sampling

1. Position patient (left lateral preferable to lithotomy) and prepare instrument tray.
2. Insert amnioscope appropriate to degree of cervical dilatation to approximate baby's scalp, withdraw introducer and attach light source.
3. Clean fetal scalp, spray with ethyl chloride (reactive hyperaemia) and apply Vaseline with a dental roll (surface tension).
4. Incise fetal scalp with a guarded blade at slight angle, wait for formation of blood droplet, apply capillary tube and collect blood.
5. Consider second sample whilst first is being analyzed. Apply pressure with cotton wool ball to ensure haemostasis.

Topics to prepare for discussion: indications and contraindications; interpretation of results.

Cervical cerclage

This technique is learnt as part of an advanced training study module in labour ward management, so you are unlikely to be asked specifically about it. However, be aware of the different techniques:

- Vaginal cerclage:
  - McDonald suture;
  - Shirodkar suture (vaginal incision, suture placed higher compared to McDonald suture);

- Abdominal cerclage (including laparoscopic).

Topics to prepare for discussion: indications; emergency cerclage.

Instrumental delivery

Ventouse delivery:

1. Thorough abdominal/pelvic examination with particular attention to position and station of head.
2. Adequate analgesia/anaesthesia (perineal, pudendal, regional).
3. Empty the bladder (do not leave indwelling catheter).
4. Place cup as near as possible to posterior fontanelle (i.e. over flexing point of occiput).
5. Activate vacuum (negative pressure initially of 0.2 kg/cm^2, check cup position and exclude incorporation of vaginal mucosa, then increase to 0.8 kg/cm^2).
6. Apply traction synchronized with maternal contractions/expulsive efforts in the plane of the birth canal (i.e. the direction of pull will change as the head descends – downward – horizontal – vertical). Maximum of three pulls recommended.
7. Support and protect the perineum with non-dominant hand as head crowns and guide mother's expulsive efforts to ensure slow, gentle delivery with minimal trauma.
8. Carefully remove the Ventouse cup after switching off vacuum.

Traction forceps delivery:

1. Thorough abdominal/pelvic examination with particular attention to position and station of head. Ensure that the sagittal suture is in the vertical plane.
2. Adequate analgesia/anaesthesia (perineal + pudendal, regional).
3. Assemble forceps to ensure correct type and they represent a 'set'.
4. Insert left blade with left hand, using right hand to guide and protect vagina. Repeat for right blade, this time using the opposite hand, and bring the handles gently together to ensure easy locking in a horizontal plane with the sagittal suture remaining in a vertical plane.
5. Apply traction synchronized with maternal contractions/expulsive efforts in the plane of the birth canal (i.e. the direction of pull will change as the head descends – downward – horizontal – vertical). Maximum of three pulls recommended.
6. Make a right mediolateral episiotomy as the perineum is being stretched, support/protect the perineum with non-dominant hand as head crowns and

guide mother's expulsive efforts to ensure slow, gentle delivery with minimal trauma.

7. Carefully remove forceps blades.

Topics to prepare for discussion: relevant obstetric definitions (i.e. pelvic diameters, relationship of presenting part to pelvis, level of instrumental delivery); conditions required for safe application of instruments; indications and contraindications; change of instruments; trial of instrumental delivery; rotational delivery – manual, Ventouse and Kielland's forceps; complications.

Caesarean section

Abdominal entry:

1. Transverse, approximately 15 cm, symmetrical lower abdominal incision (Pfannenstiel or Cohen), approximately 2 cm above the symphysis pubis (below the superior aspect of the pubic hairline ideally).
2. Incise centrally through the subcutaneous tissues and rectus sheath followed by sharp or blunt extension of incision.
3. Parietal peritoneum identified between rectus muscles, peritoneum incised and opened in a transverse plane.
4. Uterine rotation corrected manually, insert Doyen retractor and expose lower part of the uterus.
5. Elevate uterovesical peritoneum, incise transversely using scissors and push lower edge of peritoneum and attached bladder inferiorly.

Uterine entry and delivery:

1. Curved 3-cm incision into the now exposed lower uterine segment, careful entry into the uterine cavity using sharp or blunt dissection, membranes incised and fingers used bluntly to extend the incision laterally.
2. Insert hand inferiorly into the uterine cavity below the presenting part and gently elevate until presenting part appears within the uterine incision.
3. Fundal pressure applied by assistant and baby delivered.
4. Intravenous oxytocin administered by anaesthetist, placenta/membranes delivered with controlled cord traction and uterine cavity swabbed to remove any retained products of conception.

Surgical closure:*

1. Closure of uterus in double layer with continuous locking/non-locking long-acting absorbable suture, e.g. 1 Vicryl® or Polysorb® (alternatively a single layer closure).
2. Closure of rectus sheath with continuous absorbable/non-absorbable suture (e.g. 1 Vicryl® or 1 Polydioxanone [PDS®]).

3. Skin closure with fine (e.g. 2/0) absorbable (e.g. Vicryl rapide® or Monocryl®) or non-absorbable (e.g. 2/0 Proline®) subcutaneous suture.

*Peritoneal layers and fat layers do not require routine closure.

Topics to prepare for discussion: indications; classical uterine incisions; repeat caesarean sections; emergency second-stage operations; preterm delivery; oligohydramnios; abnormal lie; breech delivery; twin delivery; single vs double layer closure; high head/low head; placenta praevia; obesity; thrombo-prophylaxis; complications.

Gynaecological procedures

Vaginal hysterectomy

1. Incise and circumscribe the vaginal mucosa at the cervico-vaginal junction (most surgeons will empty the bladder and infiltrate the vaginal mucosa with saline/local anaesthetic and vasoconstrictors to reduce blood loss and help identify tissue plane).
2. Reflect the bladder from the cervix by sharp and/or blunt dissection.
3. Open the posterior peritoneum to enter the pouch of Douglas.
4. Clamp, cut and tie the uterosacral ligaments ± cardinal ligaments.
5. Open the anterior peritoneum to enter the utero-vesical space.
6. Clamp, cut and tie the uterine vessels within the broad ligament ± cardinal ligaments.
7. Deliver the uterine fundus into the vagina.
8. Clamp, cut and tie the ovarian ligament (infundibulo-pelvic ligament if salpingo-oophorectomy) and the round ligament.
9. Closure of vaginal vault, incorporating peritoneum and utero-sacral ligaments (for vault support). Commonly, a McCall culdoplasty is done (i.e. a single suture to incorporate the vaginal wall, peritoneum and utero-sacral ligaments, aimed at obliterating the posterior cul de sac).

Topics to prepare for discussion: contraindications.

Abdominal hysterectomy

There are many variations to the standard approach described below.
Abdominal entry:

1. Transverse suprapubic incision (alternatively midline abdominal incision) ~ 2–3 cm above the symphysis pubis (below the superior aspect of the pubic hairline ideally).

2. Incise centrally through the subcutaneous tissues and rectus sheath and expose the underlying parietal peritoneum by incising the median raphe (pyrimidalis if present is reflected away at this point) followed by sharp or blunt extension of incision (± reflection of the rectus sheath of the underlying muscles in a cephalad direction if greater access required).
3. Parietal peritoneum identified between rectus muscles, peritoneum incised and opened in a transverse plane.

Hysterectomy

1. Place patient in Trendelenberg position, pack away bowel and insert self-retaining retractor.
2. Uterus stabilized, round ligament clamped and cut to enter the broad ligament (ureters can be identified retroperitoneally by further dissection through the areolar tissue into the base of the broad ligament).
3. Incise the posterior leaf of the broad ligament (after identifying the ureter intra- or extra-peritoneally), clamp and transect the ovarian ligament/Fallopian tube pedicle (infunidbulo-pelvic ligament if salpingo-oophorectomy) and ligate pedicle followed by round ligament. Repeat on the other side.
4. Reflect the bladder inferiorly by incising and dissecting the anterior leaf of the broad ligament and peritoneum of the utero-vesical fold.
5. Clamp, cut and tie the uterine vessels (if subtotal hysterectomy, transect uterus below these pedicles, cauterize the cervical canal ± oversew the supravagianl cervix).
6. Clamp, cut and tie the cardinal ligaments ± uterosacral ligaments.
7. Clamp vaginal angles, transect vagina and remove uterus (alternatively enter vagina centrally first, followed by clamping and transaction of the vaginal angles). Tie vaginal angles and close vagina (continuous or interrupted sutures – alternatively leave open using a purse-string vaginal suture).

Surgical closure*

1. Closure of rectus sheath with continuous absorbable/non-absorbable suture (e.g. 1 Vicryl® or 1 Polydioxanone [PDS®]).
2. Skin closure with fine (e.g. 2/0) absorbable (e.g. Vicryl rapide® or Monocryl®) or non-absorbable (e.g. 2/0 Proline®) subcutaneous suture.

*Peritoneal layers and fat layers do not require routine closure.

Topics to prepare for discussion: route of hysterectomy (abdominal, laparoscopic, vaginal); total vs subtotal hysterectomy; complications.

Emergency gynaecological procedures

Evacuation of retained products of conception

1. Grasp the cervix with a volsellum, ask the anaesthetist to administer 5 units of intravenous oxytocin and gently dilate the cervix using graduated Hegar dilators.
2. Insert suction cannula (e.g. Karman®) of appropriate diameter to the uterine fundus and evacuate the uterine cavity using gentle rotatory and back-and-forth movements (an empty cavity is suggested by uterine contraction and 'gritty' sensation as the suction catheter abrades uterine walls. Gentle blunt curettage can be used to confirm the cavity is empty).
3. Alternatively, a blunt curette and/or polyp forceps can be used to retrieve the products of conception.

Topics to prepare for discussion: cervical prostaglandin preparation; role of antibiotics/genital tract screening; indications/contraindications for surgical ERPC; surgical ERPC for trophoblastic disease.

Bartholin's abscess ('incision and drainage')

1. Open (linear incision should be made over the medial pointing surface), drain and send pus to microbiology. Drainage should be ensured by the insertion of a gauze wick.
2. Consider treatment with appropriate antibiotics if the patient is febrile, the abscess large or there is surrounding cellulitis (the most common organisms are streptococci, *Escherichia coli*, proteus, chlamydia and gonococci).
3. Marsupialization involves incising and draining the abscess followed by suturing the edge of the infected cyst cavity to the labial skin edges using interrupted, dissolvable sutures to lay it open, reducing the chance of recurrence.

Ectopic pregnancy

1. **Salpingectomy**. The Fallopian tube containing the ectopic gestation is identified, elevated, separated from the ovary and removed by cutting and ligating the mesosalpinx and tube proximal to the products of conception. This is preferably achieved laparoscopically (using preformed 'endoloops' or energy modalities such as electrodiathermy) as surgical morbidity and the recovery time is reduced compared to laparotomy (suprapubic or midline incision).
   A partial salpingectomy removes a short section of tube containing the ectopic rather than the whole length of tube.

2. **Salpingotomy**. This involves a linear incision along the antimesenteric border of the tube over the ectopic gestation, the products of conception are removed mechanically or with suction and the bleeding points are coagulated. This technique should be reserved for managing tubal pregnancy in the presence of contralateral tubal disease and the desire for future fertility.

Topics to prepare for discussion: advantages/disadvantages of salpingectomy vs salpingotomy; when to perform laparotomy.

Example question and structured mark sheet

OSCE Q – Operative vaginal delivery ventouse (Practical competencies)

Candidate's instructions

At this station you will have 14 minutes to answer questions and demonstrate practical competencies in relation to operative vaginal delivery.

The examiner will ask you a series of questions about the practice of operative vaginal delivery and will provide you with relevant instruments as part of the structured viva.

Marks will be awarded for:

- Your ability to answer the questions about indications and techniques of operative vaginal delivery;
- Your appreciation and understanding of safety issues;
- Your knowledge and application of instrumentation.

Examiner's instructions

This is a structured viva and assessment of practical skills. At this station, the candidate will have 14 minutes to answer questions related to endoscopic surgery and demonstrate the relevant competencies. You should ask the candidate the questions on the mark sheet and provide the candidate with the ventouse devices and pelvic/fetal model as appropriate. You can prompt the candidate if necessary, but this requirement should be reflected in the marks awarded.

You should have the following equipment:

- Silicone rubber cup ('Silc cup');
- Kiwi™ OmniCup (Bird modification cup);
- Pelvic model;
- 'Fetal' doll.

Questions to be asked:
Give the candidate the two ventouse vacuum devices.

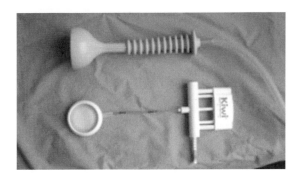

1. Ask the candidate to identify each instrument and to describe the key design differences between the devices? Then ask what fetal position and type of operative delivery they would use each device for.
2. Assuming the prerequisites for operative vaginal delivery have been satisfied, what are the specific contraindications for use of ventouse-assisted vaginal delivery?

Give the candidate the Kiwi Omnicup (Bird) and hold the model of the female pelvis and baby. Hold the doll in an occipito-posterior (OP) position.

3. Ask the candidate to describe and show you the optimal placement of the ventouse cup.

Now hold the doll in an occipito-transverse (OT) position within the female pelvic model.

4. Ask the candidate to show you and describe how they would conduct an OT ventouse delivery (assume all prerequisites of operative vaginal delivery have been met).
5. When would you abandon ventouse operative vaginal delivery?
6. If the ventouse fails, when would you apply obstetric forceps and what would you do before applying them?

Structured mark sheet

1. Ask the candidate to identify each instrument and to describe the key design differences between the devices? Then ask what fetal position and type of operative delivery they would use each device for. **[3]**

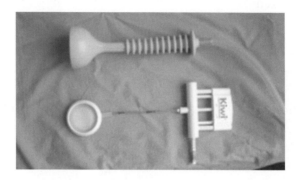

- Both ventouse devices – one silicone rubber cup and the other Kiwi™ OmniCup (Bird modification cup).
- The Kiwi™ OmniCup:
  - Modified Bird cup (low profile mushroom-shaped cup);
  - Traction + integral vacuum delivery system (foam filter, palm pump, vacuum indicator gauge and release button);
  - Sterile single use (disposable) device.
- Silicone rubber cup ('Silc-cup'):
  - Bell-shaped soft flexible silicone rubber cup;
  - Integrated vacuum (interior is lined with small projections to enable air to be evacuated) and traction shaft with moulded ridges to facilitate grip + need external suction device;
  - Reusable (autoclavable).
- Position/type of delivery:
  - The Kiwi™ OmniCup (modified Bird cup): all OA, OT and OP fetal malpositions;
  - Silicone rubber cup ('Silc-cup'): OA position and outlet (vertex) deliveries.

0   1   2   3

2. Assuming the prerequisites for operative vaginal delivery have been satisfied, what are the specific contraindications for use of ventouse assisted vaginal delivery? **[2]**

- Face presentation.
- Marked active bleeding from a fetal blood sampling site.
- Gestation < 34 weeks.

0   1   2

3. Ask the candidate to describe and show you the optimal placement of the ventouse cup. [1]

Midline over the occiput covering the posterior fontanelle [middle of cup over the flexion point of the fetal head (3 cm forward of posterior fontanelle)].

0   1

4. Ask the candidate to show you and describe how they would conduct an OT ventouse delivery (assume all prerequisites of operative vaginal delivery have been met). [6]

- Apply lubricant to the outside of the cup (e.g. Hibitane cream).
- Atraumatic vaginal insertion (part labia and wait for uterine relaxation) over the occiput.
- Take the negative pressure to 0.2 kg/cm^2 and check that no vaginal tissue is caught under the cup.
- Take the negative pressure to 0.8 kg/cm^2.
- Gentle traction beginning with the peak of each contraction/maternal effort (midwife and/or you coach the mother) in the plane of the pelvis (pelvic axis) for the duration of the contraction.
- One hand should rest on the cup (to prevent detachment and gauge descent ± use fingers to promote head flexion) and the other hand applies traction.
- No requirement for routine episiotomy (no increase in presenting diameter cf forceps). Use as for standard obstetric indications.
- As the head crowns, change the angle of traction through 90° and control delivery of head [protect perineum with hand, mother to stop pushing ('pant')].
- Check neck for cord – loosen, take off neck and deliver shoulders with next contraction/maternal effort after restitution with external rotation and lateral flexion. Deliver placenta (active 3rd stage ± elective oxytocin infusion – risk PPH).
- Careful vaginal/perineal/rectal examination and repair episiotomy/tears [check baby's head for significant chignon (or cephalohaematoma) and explain to parents 'egg-head' to be expected – should resolve in 2–4 days].
- Documentation (and review prior to discharge).

0   1   2   3   4   5   6

5. When would you abandon ventouse operative vaginal delivery? [2]

- No evidence of progressive decent with each pull (the head, not just the scalp, should descend with each pull).
- Delivery not imminent following three pulls/contractions (of a correctly applied instrument by an experienced operator).
- > 15 minutes elapsed since application of instrument.
- More than one cup detachment (an experienced operator should be summoned after one detachment for reapplication if feasible).
- Woman withdraws consent.

0   1   2

6. If the ventouse fails, when would you apply obstetric forceps and what would you do before applying them? [2]

- Prior to application:
  - Explain situation to patient/couple;
  - Call for help if senior help available and feasible;
  - Re-examine the patient to recheck fetal position, station (is the head engaged?, i.e. is the caput felt below the ischial spines?);
  - Checks for signs of fetal distress (CTG, FHR) – if present reconsider;
  - Careful reflection (only use sequential forceps judiciously, avoid if possible, abandon if not straightforward application or descent with one pull of forceps).
- Only use sequential obstetric forceps when failure with the ventouse occurs because of inadequate traction/vacuum. Specifically:
  - Consider following failure to gain adequate suction due to excessive caput or leaking equipment in a baby presenting by the vertex below the ischial spines;
  - Consider following cup detachment and failure to gain adequate suction on reapplication of cup after progressive decent with ventouse and fetal head (not caput) visible without parting the labia (outlet delivery);
  - Consider following incorrect placement of ventouse cup by an inexperienced operator which explains failure.

0   1   2

Global score [4]

0   1   2   3   4

Total: /20

7

Emergencies

The ability to manage emergency situations is integral to the competent practice of O&G. Medical emergencies can be stressful at the best of times, but this is particularly true in the field of obstetrics where most acute, life-threatening events tend to occur. This is because in obstetrics you are generally dealing with young, otherwise healthy women and their babies. The MRCOG Part 2 allows examiners to evaluate the ability of candidates to think clearly and act appropriately in the acute situation where the life of the mother or baby may be at stake. For the purpose of the part 2 examination, we would recommend preparing and practising commonly encountered emergency situations, in simulated 'emergency drills' if possible. There are some excellent postgraduate courses, e.g. The MOET course (Managing Obstetric Emergencies and Trauma): attendance at such a course would be ideal preparation and give confidence to the part 2 candidate.

This chapter gives guidance on how to tackle these stations successfully and provides suggested summaries for revising. The management of less common obstetric emergencies, medical emergencies and trauma is beyond the scope of this revision book.

How to approach the 'emergency' station

Digest the question/scenario before answering

Your aim is to not only to provide the correct information but also to do so in a logical, systematic manner to demonstrate confidence in your abilities to the examiner. This is unlikely to be achieved by the nervous, impetuous candidate who 'rushes in' with an answer without allowing due time for reflection.

Adopt a structured approach

You will normally be presented with a brief clinical scenario, but to aid your initial rapid clinical assessment do not forget to seek further important information from the midwife (and patient if appropriate) if the underlying clinical situation is unclear. Appropriate questioning will obviously depend upon the particular clinical scenario but may include questions such as: 'Does the patient have any medical problems?' (in the case of unexplained collapse); 'What is the estimated blood loss?' or 'Is the placenta low lying?' (in the case of haemorrhage); 'Have there been any antenatal problems?' (in the case of fetal distress). Such questioning should however take place simultaneously with 'ABC' resuscitation: i.e. **A**irway, **B**reathing and ventilation, and **C**irculation, with aggressive volume replacement and control of haemorrhage (if present). Make a decision at this point about the need to 'call for help', which means having additional staff immediately available on the labour ward, as well as informing or acquiring senior (consultant) input.

'ABC' resuscitation

- Involve the anaesthetist to manage the airway, breathing (supplementary oxygen, e.g. 8 L/min) and ventilation.
- Mange the circulation with a minimum of two large-calibre intravenous lines (e.g. 16 gauge upwards).
- Take bloods, which generally means a FBC, coagulation screen, U&Es and cross-match* in the case of haemorrhage. In the case of unexplained collapse/altered consciousness take a blood glucose, urates, LFTs and pregnancy test as appropriate.
- Replace circulating volume rapidly if blood loss suspected, using warmed crystalloid/colloid initially and blood/blood products when available.
- Monitoring (insert urinary catheter with hourly bag; continuous pulse/BP/ECG/oximeter monitoring; consider arterial/CVP lines).
- Stop the bleeding (approach depends upon the cause – see specific scenario summaries).

*O negative blood can be acquired immediately in acute haemorrhage with cardiovascular compromise or, if the blood group is known, then type-specific blood ordered (available in < 10 minutes) in addition to a request for fully cross-matched blood.

If the scenario is an antenatal/perinatal obstetric emergency, then once maternal resuscitation has begun, assess the wellbeing and viability of the fetus (i.e. electronic fetal monitoring ± ultrasound if available). Clearly, if the scenario is one of fetal distress in an otherwise well mother, then 'ABCs' are not required and you should move directly to assessment of the fetus and diagnosing the cause of the fetal problem. Once resuscitation has begun (and the patient's condition is stabilizing), then review the medical history and perform an abdominal/pelvic examination ± systemic examination as appropriate to arrive at a probable diagnosis (e.g. placental abruption, cord prolapse, pre-eclampsia/eclampsia). Finally, specific treatment should be instituted according to the diagnosis (e.g. uterotonic agents, antibiotics, delivery) and response to treatment evaluated on a continuous basis. Clear, contemporary documentation is key, both as a matter of good practice but also from the medicolegal standpoint. The overall approach is summarized below.

Structured approach to managing emergencies in O&G

- Rapid assessment of situation + communicate
- 'ABC' resuscitation
- Call for help (if appropriate)
- Assess fetal wellbeing and viability (if appropriate)
- Make a diagnosis
- Institute specific treatment
- Evaluation of response
- Documentation

Provide the information in the context of the real life clinical setting

You will have encountered most situations in clinical practice. It is useful to 'picture' these past experiences in your mind to help assemble your thoughts in the correct sequence. Examiners will quickly spot the candidate who appears to be 'reciting from the textbook of obstetric emergencies' rather than relying on past clinical experience when describing their approach.

Remember to delegate and use facilities

The effective management of medical emergencies requires a multidisciplinary team approach. The question may 'provide' you with 'available staff' but, if not, it is reasonable to assume that you have resident midwives, healthcare assistants, porters, an SHO in obstetrics and an anaesthetic registrar, as well as available consultant staff in O&G, anaesthetics and haematology. In addition, most units have high dependency unit (HDU) beds on labour ward or available HDU/ITU beds elsewhere in the hospital. The good candidate will effectively delegate tasks according to experience and clinical competencies (see Chapter 9).

Emergency summaries – obstetric emergencies

Pre-eclampsia/eclampsia

- Communicate.
- ABC (± CVP/arterial lines).
- Diagnosis (examination, FBC, U&Es, urate, coagulation screen, G&S, MSU).
- Control seizures ($MgSO_4$).
- Control hypertension (IV labetalol or hydralazine).
- Deliver.

Massive obstetric haemorrhage

- Communicate.
- ABC (± CVP/arterial lines).
- Replace circulating volume/blood/blood products.
- Diagnosis (examination, FBC ± Kleihauer, coagulation screen, cross-match).
- Stop bleeding.

Uterine atony

- Empty uterus + bimanual compression.
- Uterotonic agents [oxytocin 5 units IV, ergometrine 500 mg IV, prostaglandins, e.g. misoprostol 800 mg PR, carboprost 250 mg IM; antifibrinolytics aprotonin 2 000 000 units, tranexamic acid 1 g IV; recombinant factor VIIa 90 mg/kg IV (discuss with haematologist)].
- Uterine tamponade (packing or Rusch balloon).
- Laparotomy (uterine sparing – internal iliac artery/uterine artery ligation, uterine compression sutures, e.g. B-Lynch brace suture; hysterectomy).
- Interventional radiology (arterial embolization).

Disseminated intravascular coagulopathy

Clotting factors (FFP/cryoprecipitate and platelets).

Genital tract trauma

- Repair of uterine/genital tract injury.
- Topical fibrin.

Signs of hypovolaemia

- Tachycardia
- Hypotension*
- Cold, clammy, pale skin (especially peripheries)
- Poor urine output
- Altered conscious level

*Hypotension (this is a relatively late sign associated with significant blood loss as the cardiovascular system in most young women will compensate initially, such that up to 35% of their circulating blood volume may be lost before the blood pressure falls)

Antepartum haemorrhage

- Communicate.
- Resuscitation as for 'massive obstetric haemorrhage' if major APH with haemodynamic shock.
- Diagnosis [examination – abdominal (abruption), speculum (local cause), USS to exclude placenta praevia (no VE unless this is excluded), FBC ± Kleihauer (give anti-D 500 IU if Rhesus negative), coagulation screen, cross-match].
- Assess fetal wellbeing.
- *Placental abruption.* Deliver fetus* (C/S vs IOL) if fetal or maternal compromise.
- *Placenta praevia.* Deliver fetus* (C/S) if fetal or maternal compromise.
*Threshold for delivery will depend upon gestation.

Uterine inversion

- Communicate.
- ABC (± CVP/arterial lines).

- Replace circulating volume/blood/blood products.
- Diagnosis (vaginal examination, FBC, coagulation screen, cross-match).
- Replace inversion as soon as possible (do not remove placenta until uterus is replaced):
  - Manual replacement;
  - Hydrostatic repositioning (O'Sullivans's technique);
  - Consider uterine relaxation to facilitate [e.g. terbutaline, volatile agent (GA)];
  - Surgical replacement (laparotomy).

Cord prolapse

- Communicate.
- Diagnosis (VE).
- Assess fetal wellbeing (EFM).
- Relieve pressure on umbilical cord:
  - Manual elevation + knee-chest or Trendelenburg positioning;
  - Bladder filling (Foley catheter + 500 ml Normal saline);
- Caesarean section.
- Instrumental delivery if fully dilated.

Shoulder dystocia

- Communicate.
- Position patient (draw buttocks to edge of bed; lie supine and hyperflex hips – McRobert's manoeuvre).
- Consider episiotomy.
- Suprapubic pressure + traction.
- Manoeuvres (deliver posterior arm/shoulder; internal rotatory manoeuvres, e.g. Woods' screw).
- Change of position (on all fours – Gaskin manoeuvre).
- Extreme measures (Zavanelli manoeuvre, cleidotomy; symphysiotomy).
- Examine genital tract for trauma and repair.

Twin pregnancy

- Deliver twin I.
- Check lie (clinical/USS) and FHR twin II (EFM).
- Transverse lie (1st line = ECV; 2nd line IPV + assisted breech delivery).
- ARM with contraction when presenting part in pelvis.
- Aim for NVD (instrumental delivery if delay or fetal distress).

Additional considerations for twin delivery

- Inform anaesthetist/paediatrician/neonatal unit
- Epidural (potential need for uterine manipulations)
- Consider transfer to theatre (particularly if twin II is not longitudinal)
- Oxytocin infusion (10 IU in 40 ml Hartmann's solution) ready for second stage if no contractions within 5–10 min
- Oxytocin infusion (40 IU in 40 ml Hartmann's solution) ready for third stage (increased risk of PPH)

Vaginal breech delivery

- Consider epidural (potential need for vaginal manipulations).
- Await breech descent to pelvic floor before maternal pushing.
- Await spontaneous delivery of breech ± episiotomy (once anus visible over fourchette; note: 'hands off').
- Ensure sacrum rotates anteriorly and deliver extended hips by flexion at knee joint.
- Bring down loop of cord and wrap towel around baby's trunk to keep warm.
- Deliver anterior arm [once anterior shoulder scapula visible – run finger over shoulder to elbow and 'sweep' out by flexion and traction at elbow joint. Repeat for other shoulder (which will rotate anteriorly); Lovsett's manoeuvre for hyperextended/nuchal arm].
- Delivery of head:
    - Mauriceau–Smellie–Veit manoeuvre;
    - Burns Marshall manoeuvre;
    - Forceps.

Emergency summaries – gynaecological emergencies

Miscarriage and haemorrhage with haemodynamic shock

- Communicate.
- ABC.
- Diagnosis [examination and remove products of conception from cervical canal (resolves vaso-vagal reaction), FBC, coagulation screen, G&S].
- Syntometrine® IM/IV (oxytocin 5 IU + ergometrine 0.5 mg).
- Transfer to theatre.
- Surgical ERPC.

Ruptured ectopic pregnancy with haemodynamic shock

- Communicate.
- ABC (± CVP/arterial lines – do not delay surgical intervention).
- Diagnosis (examination, urinary pregnancy test, FBC, coagulation screen, G&S).
- Transfer to theatre.
- Laparotomy.

Example question and structured mark sheet

OSCE Q – Shoulder dystocia (Practical competencies)

Candidate's instructions

At this station you will have 14 minutes to answer questions and demonstrate practical competencies in relation to management of an obstetric emergency delivery.

You are the SpR on call for obstetrics and the emergency alarm sounds on labour ward with an instruction to go to Room 7 immediately. You arrive to find that the baby's head has been delivered, but the midwife cannot deliver the shoulders.

The examiner will ask you to discuss and demonstrate, using the pelvis and doll provided, how you would manage this situation.

Marks will be awarded for:

- Demonstrable practical skills and proficiency;
- Understanding of the manoeuvres available, their sequence and their rationale;
- Other knowledge relevant to this obstetric emergency.

Examiner's instructions

You should ask the candidate to demonstrate the relevant manoeuvres in the management of this obstetric emergency, and then ask the questions in the order they appear on your mark sheet. You can prompt the candidate if necessary, but this requirement should be reflected in the marks awarded.

You should have the following equipment:

- 'Fetal' doll;
- Pelvic model.

Questions to be asked:

1. Ask the candidate to take you through the steps in managing this obstetric emergency and demonstrate the relevant obstetric manoeuvres in a logical sequence using the doll provided. You should hold the pelvis as required.

Once the candidate has finished, ask them the following questions.

2. How does shoulder dystocia happen?
3. What factors may be associated with shoulder dystocia?
4. What pre-emptive action to prevent shoulder dystocia would you consider in a diabetic woman with a BMI of 35 and a 4.3 kg baby?

Structured mark sheet

1. Ask the candidate to take you through the steps in managing this obstetric emergency and demonstrate the relevant obstetric manoeuvres in a logical sequence using the doll provided. **[10]**

- Call for help. Expertise is important – senior obstetrician, midwives/ ancillary staff, anaesthetist, paediatrician (SpR upwards). Minutes count in baby's prognosis if asphyxia/trauma.
- Take bottom of the bed and draw the buttocks to the edge. This allows optimal lateral flexion.
- Consider episiotomy:
  - Allows room for internal manoeuvres (access to sacral hollow);
  - Reduce likelihood of vaginal lacerations.
- McRobert's manoeuvre – maximum flexion, abduction and external rotation of the hips (manual, not lithotomy poles) ± moderate traction. This straightens the sacrum relative to the lumbar vertebrae, leading to upward rotation of the pelvis, freeing the impacted shoulder + also increases the uterine pressure and amplitude of contractions.
- Suprapubic pressure + moderate traction – heel of hand applies constant or rocking pressure (for 30 s) (in a downward and lateral direction) to the posterior aspect of the shoulder. This adducts, reducing the bisacromial diameter, and internally rotates the anterior shoulder into the oblique pelvic diameter; it should then slip underneath the symphysis pubis with the aid of routine traction.

- Deliver posterior arm and shoulder – operator's hand is passed up to the fetal axilla, gentle traction applied posteriorly and the shoulder hooked down bringing the posterior arm into reach. Then apply backward pressure on the cubital fossa to disimpact the arm. Hold the fetal hand and sweep it across the chest and face and out of the vagina:
  - More room in sacral hollow (thus go for posterior shoulder);
  - Access the shoulder and disengage the fetal arm to enable delivery.
- Internal rotational manoeuvres: aim is to rotate the shoulders into an oblique diameter or by a full 180°:
  1. Wood's screw – insert the fingers of the opposite hand vaginally so that you approach the posterior shoulder from the front of the fetus, aiming to rotate the shoulder towards the symphysis pubis;
  2. Reverse screw – place fingers on the posterior shoulder from behind the fetus and rotate in the opposite direction;
  3. Rubin II – insert the fingertips behind the anterior shoulder and push it forward towards the fetal chest (adducting the shoulders and rotating the bisacromial diameter into the oblique). This manoeuvre can be combined with the Wood's screw to rotate the shoulders through 180°.
- Change of position – roll over onto all fours ('Gaskin' manoeuvre). This increases the AP diameter of the inlet and facilitates other manoeuvres (e.g. delivery of posterior (with respect to the maternal pelvis) shoulder).
- Extreme measures:
  - Zavanelli manoeuvre (cephalic replacement by rotating/flexing/re-inserting fetal head into the vagina followed by caesarean section). This bypasses pelvic outlet;
  - Symphysiotomy (incomplete midline cut through the cartilaginous symphyseal joint). This increases the space available to facilitate delivery of the shoulders;
  - Cleidotomy. This allows excess adduction and manipulation of the fetal shoulder and arm.
- Do not:
  - Apply fundal pressure;
  - Encourage maternal pushing efforts unless shoulder displacement has been achieved.

0   1   2   3   4   5   6   7   8   9   10

Once the candidate has finished, ask them the following questions.

2. How does shoulder dystocia happen? [2]

Failure of the shoulders to rotate into the AP diameter as they traverse the pelvic cavity. The posterior shoulder usually enters the pelvic cavity while the anterior shoulder remains hooked behind the symphysis pubis. In more severe forms, both shoulders do cross the pelvic brim.

0   1   2

3. What factors may be associated with shoulder dystocia? [2]

- Antenatal factors:
    - Previous shoulder dystocia;
    - Macrosomia;
    - Diabetes mellitus;
    - Maternal BMI > 30 kg/m^2;
    - Induction of labour.
- Intrapartum factors:
    - Prolonged first stage of labour;
    - Secondary arrest;
    - Prolonged second stage of labour;
    - Oxytocin augmentation;
    - Assisted vaginal delivery.

0   1   2

4. What pre-emptive action to prevent shoulder dystocia would you consider in a diabetic woman with a BMI of 35 and a 4.3 kg baby? [2]

- Consider caesarean section.
- Not IOL unless for diabetic indications [there is no evidence that it reduces the maternal or neonatal morbidity from shoulder dystocia (although incidence slightly reduced)].
- Experienced obstetrician (SpR upwards) should be available on labour ward during the second stage of labour.

0   1   2

Global score [4]

0   1   2   3   4

Total: /20

8

Structured oral examination (viva)

The structured oral examination or 'viva' is a station where you will be asked a set of ordered questions by the examiner. Such stations may be integrated into 'clinical management'- or 'data interpretation'-type stations or they may be stand-alone. Many candidates will be familiar with viva examinations from their undergraduate days or job interviews. Even if you are not, the station format is straightforward and this form of oral exam allows you an opportunity to demonstrate your knowledge and ability to communicate. A suggested, successful approach to these stations is outlined below.

Demeanour

- Greet and/or introduce yourself. Stay calm and be pleasant.
- Be attentive – this means maintain a good posture (do not slouch) and eye contact, and, despite your nerves, aim to look interested and smile!
- Stay focused throughout, maintain your self-confidence and composure even if you feel the interview is not going well.
- Do not become argumentative or allow the discussion to become heated, even if you feel the examiner is unreasonably critical.
- Do not be alarmed if the examiner finishes questioning you before the bell goes. You have probably done well. Simply sit quietly unless the examiner wants to engage you in conversation. Resist the temptation to ask: 'How have I done?'
- Thank the examiner when leaving the station.

Answering questions

Listen carefully to the question, and answer directly. It is surprisingly common for candidates to answer a different, often unrelated question! Indeed, this tendency is not limited to exam candidates, but also to trainees or medical students usually as a result of becoming 'flustered' when they are 'put on the spot' by senior colleagues in day-to-day clinical practice settings. To an examiner this can be very irritating, especially when they are trying to follow a prepared format. Another annoyance to examiners is the 'parrot-like' repetition of their questions out of habit.

Follow instructions exactly – if a short answer is requested, keep your answer short. If more detail is desired, give a longer response. Try to answer the question as it is posed, remembering that you are engaged in an academic conversation.

Do not interrupt the examiner. Wait until they finish the question before you start to answer. Indeed, a good approach is to pause briefly after each question is asked. This allows you to take a moment to compose yourself, formulate some thoughts and decide where to begin.

Do not answer questions with just a 'yes' or 'no'. It is difficult to explore a candidate's knowledge if they are somewhat monosyllabic. You should demonstrate your in-depth knowledge by expanding on your answer. When you do this, however, it is important to ensure that you have clearly answered the set question, that you are confident of the additional, related information you are now providing and you remain concise (i.e. do not bore the examiner with a prepared speech!). Stick to two or three key points or examples.

If you have not understood the question, seek clarification by asking the examiner to rephrase it, or alternatively give your interpretation and ask if that is what was meant. If you still do not understand the question, then it is better to admit it than to try and bluff. Do not 'ramble' if you have understood the question but do not know an answer. In such circumstances ask for clarification if appropriate, but if you are sure you cannot answer the question then admit this, i.e. state directly that you do not know the answer. This allows the examiner to rephrase the question, which may help you formulate an answer, or move to the next question where you may score marks rather than wasting time 'digging a deep hole' that you cannot climb out of!

Do not carry 'baggage'. Remember that each new question represents a new opportunity to gain marks, so put a previous bad question to the back of your mind. There will be plenty of time to ruminate about this later, once the exam is over, but it will not help you in the exam and indeed will have a detrimental effect.

Come across as an 'intelligent listener', i.e. you are more likely to convey a good impression if you appear attentive and interested in what the examiner has to say. This is especially important if you have failed to answer a question correctly, as your apparent willingness to learn from the examiner will be looked upon favourably.

Engage the examiner. Although the emphasis of these structured oral tests is on your providing answers similar to those on the examiner's structured mark sheet, when a viva is going well, the interaction with the examiner is often a two-way process involving you talking *and* listening and maybe even discussing issues and providing opinions. A *viva voce* examination, say when presenting a university thesis, will set out to interrogate the candidate and test the limits of their knowledge. In this professional examination, this is not the aim, so if the examiner goes 'off message' and starts asking more dynamic, difficult, open-ended questions, then do not panic. It is likely the examiner thinks you are a good candidate and they are filling the time and enjoying the interaction.

Learn when to 'stop talking'! If the examiner identifies an area of weakness, concede the point gracefully. However, in clinical medicine there is often no absolutely 'right' or 'wrong' answer, so be prepared to justify your answer. If the examiner challenges your position, then reconsider your answer, but if you still believe that your initial response was a good one, then present your case firmly but in a courteous manner.

Example question and structured mark sheet

OSCE Q – Obesity and pregnancy (Viva, management)

Candidate's instructions

At this station you will have 14 minutes to answer questions about obstetric care.

This is a structured viva. The examiner will ask you a series of questions about issues relating to the management of obese women in pregnancy.

Marks will be awarded for:

Your ability to answer questions about the obstetric care of obese patients.

Examiner's instructions

At this station, the candidate will have 14 minutes to discuss the obstetric management of an obese woman. You should ask the candidate the questions in the order they appear on your mark sheet.

Questions to be asked:

1. How would you define obesity?
2. Obesity is considered a risk factor for pregnancy. What obstetric complications are associated with obesity?
3. What additional antenatal care would you arrange for a nulliparous 27-year-old woman with a BMI of 44 kg/m^2 who you are seeing at a booking antenatal clinic appointment?
4. This woman (BMI 44) requires an emergency caesarean section for a deep transverse arrest causing failure to progress in the second stage of labour. It is 02:00 and your consultant is at home. What intra- and post-operative problems would you anticipate and how would you minimize these?
5. You have difficulty delivering the impacted fetal head. What do you do to aid delivery of the baby?

Structured mark sheet

1. How would you define obesity? [1]
BMI $\geq$ 35 kg/m^2 at first contact.

0   1

2. Obesity is considered a risk factor for pregnancy. What obstetric complications are associated with obesity? [3]

- Antenatal:
  - Gestational diabetes;
  - Hypertension, pre-eclampsia;
  - Abnormal fetal growth: either macrosomia or IUGR;
  - Sleep apnoea;
  - Undiagnosed fetal anomaly.
- Intrapartum:
  - Failure to progress in labour;
  - Shoulder dystocia;
  - Difficulties monitoring fetal heart;
  - Inadequate analgesia;

- Emergency caesarean section;
- Technically difficult caesarean section, with associated increased morbidity and mortality;
- Anaesthetic risks;
- Other theatre risks – positioning/moving of the patient difficult, compromised safe use of equipment, such as lithotomy stirrups, operating tables.
- Postpartum:
  - Wound infections post operative delivery;
  - Thromboembolic events;
  - Postnatal depression.

0   1   2   3

3. What additional antenatal care would you arrange for a nulliparous 27-year-old woman with a BMI of 44 kg/m^2 who you are seeing at a booking antenatal clinic appointment? [5]

- Consultant-led care if BMI > 35.
- Glucose tolerance test (GTT) at 26 weeks to check the development of gestational diabetes.
- Encourage healthy eating and offer an appointment with a dietitian.
- Obstetric/medical risk factors related to the obesity (as outlined above) need to be discussed with the woman, and documented in a frank but sensitive way.
- Consider USS scans for fetal growth ± wellbeing (fetal weight, liquor volume and umbilical artery Doppler studies) in the third trimester (e.g. 28–34 weeks) as it can be difficult to estimate growth from palpation alone in obese women.
- Increase frequency of antenatal clinic appointments (hospital and community) due to the increased risk of pregnancy complications in this group of women (e.g. schedule at least 2 weekly from 28 weeks, and weekly from 36 weeks). Blood pressure should be checked with an appropriately sized cuff at each visit.
- Refer for an anaesthetic assessment regardless of the planned mode of delivery (e.g. between 28 and 34 weeks for most women). The woman should be re-weighed (feasibility of obstetric operating tables, etc).
- Arrange social service support, psychiatric input, etc, if social disadvantage, domestic violence, mental illness, etc, associated with obesity.

0   1   2   3   4   5

4. This woman (BMI 44) requires an emergency caesarean section for a deep transverse arrest causing failure to progress in the second stage of labour. It is 02:00 and your consultant is at home. What intra- and post-operative problems would you anticipate and how would you minimize these? [5]

- Difficulty with moving and positioning the patient. Ensure adequate staffing, appropriate weight-bearing equipment, e.g. operative table, extra assistance.
- Difficult anaesthesia. Ensure Obstetric SpR has discussed the case with their on-call consultant and asked for assistance (two anaesthetists preferable) if deemed necessary (especially if they cannot gain regional access).
- Difficult surgical access (fat, patient cannot lie flat for anaesthesia). Extra assistance (ideally senior), large Pfannensteil incision (midline rarely required to access uterus, but consider if other risk factors, e.g. adhesions from previous surgery), careful abdominal entry to ensure adequate access prior to incising the uterus.
- Wound infection. Good surgical technique (careful tissue handling, haemostasis) and use interrupted skin sutures/staples (reduce collection/ abscess). Use of broad-spectrum antibiotics intrapartum and consider postpartum. Regular review (daily).
- Venous thromboembolism. Keep well hydrated, use of intraoperative pneumatic compression stockings, administer prophylactic postpartum anticoagulant, e.g. Dalteparin (Fragmin) 5000 IU SC to upper thigh, every 24 hours (first dose to be administered no sooner than 4 hours postoperatively and no later than 24 hours postoperatively. Treatment is to be continued for a minimum of 4 days). Consider use of postpartum TED stockings.

0   1   2   3   4   5

5. You have difficulty delivering the impacted fetal head. What do you do to aid delivery of the baby? [2]

Methods to facilitate extraction of the impacted head:

- 'Push' method. Place patient in the Whitmore ('frog') position and push the deeply engaged head upwards through the vagina out of the pelvis. This manoeuvre can be done by the operator or, more usually, an assistant.
- 'Pull' method ('reverse breech'):
  - Introduce your hand through the LUS incision and up towards the upper segment, grasp the fetal legs and extract the fetus by the breech;

- LUS transverse incision may need to be adapted into an inverted T or J incision;
- ± Uterine relaxation [inhalational agent (GA)/β-mimetic, e.g. terbutaline];
- (Ventouse delivery has been reported).
- (Call consultant).

0   1   2

Global score [4]

0   1   2   3   4

Total: /20

9

Prioritization and ward rounds

Prioritization questions can take various forms, but the two commonest are prioritization on the delivery suite and of a gynaecological operating list. These questions are divided into two parts: the first 15 minutes are allocated to planning and preparing your answer in the preparatory stations; the second half is when you present your answer to the examiner and pick up your marks.

These questions can assess a number of issues:

1. Your skills at prioritization;
2. Your skills in organization;
3. Your efficient and effective 'deployment' of staff;
4. Your ability to deal with multiple tasks at a given time;
5. Your ability to provide an effective handover;
6. Your appreciation of your own limits (*'I will call the consultant from the clinic'*).

No wonder, then, that prioritization stations are very popular in the OSCE: a prioritization station of some description appearing in your exam is almost a certainty and preparing for them is easy.

Prioritization on a delivery suite

Every time you are on-call for the delivery suite, insist that you do the handover. Imagine that you are in the exam when you stand in front of the delivery suite patient board; do not take more than 15 minutes in planning your handover, and complete your handover itself within 15 minutes, thus emulating the exam conditions. Seek feedback from your colleagues, specifically on your prioritization and use of available staff.

Delivery suite prioritization can be approached as follows:

- In your preparatory station, go through every case in order. Put down your thoughts on the sheet of paper on which your 'delivery suite board' is printed (rather than wasting time copying the details into your notepad).
- Categorize the cases. You need to have a system that works for you. Some of you will categorize the cases as 'high, medium, low'; others may use 'urgent, semi-urgent, routine'; yet others may use the 'plus' signs to denote urgency (+++, ++, +, 0), with '0' indicating 'routine'. It does not matter which system you use; what matters is that you adopt one system now (if you have not already) and stick with it.
- Once you have categorized patients by their priority status, list the tasks which need to be done, and assign your staff appropriately.
- Remember safety is paramount. Thus, if there is a reasonable need to call the consultant from a clinic or some other engagement, do not hesitate to do this. However, if you call in your consultant or additional staff whenever a patient sneezes, this is likely to earn you the irritation of the examiner (who is after all very likely to be a practising clinician who gets called in by juniors appropriately and inappropriately) and may reflect on your marks.
- It is usual to present the urgent cases first, and we think this approach is good practice. However, there are marks for each case on your delivery suite board (even for the 'routine care' ones), and thus once you have addressed the urgent cases, it is important that you go through the rest of the patients on the board, case by case.
- If you are making operative decisions, particularly ones which would necessitate an entry into the theatre (e.g. a caesarean section or trial of instrument delivery in theatre), you are expected to discuss this with the consultant.
- Do not forget hidden treasures such as your anaesthetist! For instance, they may be the ideal person to review a postoperative woman with pre-eclampsia who is being managed in the high dependency unit.
- Do not hesitate to switch midwives. For example, if a specific midwife is skilled in intravenous cannulation or repairing episiotomies, then switching of midwives may be necessary to the efficient management of the delivery suite.

Prioritization of a gynaecological operating list

Many of the principles addressed above apply to this task also. In addition, the candidate is expected to assess:

1. The appropriateness of the operations being proposed. (Does the patient need an operation? If so, is this the ideal operation?)
2. The appropriateness of the venue (outpatient procedure, daycase surgery, inpatient surgery, surgery in a tertiary centre, e.g. a cancer centre).
3. Any specific special needs (e.g. bowel preparation before extensive endometriosis surgery, appropriate preoperative investigations and anaesthetic assessment in those patients with medical conditions, home support for the elderly).
4. Priority (routine, soon or urgent: routine used to be regarded as within 6 months, soon as within 12 weeks and urgent as within 4 weeks, although these priority terms are likely to acquire a different meaning with the national 18-week patient pathway initiative).

If necessary, do not hesitate to cancel an operation, particularly when the indication is inappropriate. Furthermore, pay particular attention to aspects of preoperative care, such as assessment by anaesthetists, or review by haematologists, or need to arrange special investigations such as an MRI or CT scan.

The labour ward is the commonest 'prioritization' setting for questions in the MRCOG Part 2. However, do not be fazed if settings such as acute gynaecology on call, triaging waiting lists or pre-/post-operative ward rounds are used to test prioritization and delegation, as the basic principles remain the same.

Example questions and structured mark sheet

Example 1: OSCE Q – Delivery suite prioritization (Prioritization, management)

Candidate's instructions

You are the labour ward on-call registrar, who has come to take handover at 8.30 am from the night staff. Attached you will find the details of 10 women on the labour ward board.

The following staff are on the labour ward with you:

- An SHO with 4 months experience in O&G
- An anaesthetic SpR
- Five midwifes (BMW, SU, AK, DE, SL): BMW is in charge; BMW, SU and AK can suture; all five can insert IV lines.

The on-call consultant is conducting SpR interviews, and would prefer not be interrupted unless this is necessary.

TABLE 9.1

Room	Name	Gestation	Parity	Liquor	Epidural	Synto	Comment	MW
1	Taylor	37w	3	Intact	No	No	Undiagnosed breech; 5 cm at 7.30 am	SU
2	Muto	T+10	3 (LSCS X1)	Clear	No	No	Trial of vaginal delivery; 5 cm at 4.00 am; FBS at 4 am – pH 7.27	BMW
3	Smith	37	1	Intact	–	–	Awaiting ECV; NB needs consent please	–
4	Kaur	37, Twins (DCDA)	0	Intact	Yes	No	IVF pregnancy; Ceph/Ceph; 4 cm dilated; mild PET	AK
5	Dillon	29	1	–	–	–	Abdo pain for 3 days – Dr to see please	–
6	Vinci	39	1	Mec	No	No	Transferred from Birth Centre (mw unit) at 6 am at 6 cm (as Mec)	SL
7	Said	41	7	–	–	–	Quick delivery; small tear – awaiting suturing	DE
8	Patel	34	0	Intact	Yes	Y (post-partum regime)	Delivery by CS for severe PET at 2:00 am. Good urine output	AK
9	Surya	39	1	Clear	Yes	No	4 cm at 4 am; 8 cm at 8 am	SU
10	Kuku	40	2	Clear	No	N	Fully and Pushing since 7.00 am	BMW

Read the board, and decide:

1. What tasks need to be done?
2. What order should they be done in?
3. Who should do them?

At the next station, you will discuss the board with an examiner.

Marks will be awarded for:

Your ability to prioritize and manage the labour ward effectively and safely.

Examiner's instructions

Candidates have 14 minutes to explain the following:

- The tasks that need doing on the delivery suite.
- The order in which they should be done.
- The staff they would allocate to each task.

Marks should be awarded according to the structured mark sheet provided.

Structured mark sheet and model answers

Room 1	0	1	2	3	4
Room 2	0	1	2	3	4
Room 3	0	1	2	3	4
Room 4	0	1	2	3	4
Room 5	0	1	2	3	4
Room 6	0	1	2	3	4
Room 7	0	1	2	3	4
Room 8	0	1	2	3	4
Room 9	0	1	2	3	4
Room 10	0	1	2	3	4

Gross mark: $/40 \times \frac{1}{2}$

Total: $/20$

TABLE 9.2

Room	Name	What needs doing	Priority	Who will do it?
1	Taylor	Needs urgent review re mode of delivery. Recommend epidural	+++	You
2	Muto	Needs assessment of progress; review of CTG; and + FBS	++	Send in BMW – followed by you after RM1 – If BMW concerned about CTG (+++), call consultant
3	Smith	Non-urgent; needs USS to ascertain presentation; ensure bloods results in notes and NBM; consent	0	You (when free); SHO can help you
4	Kaur	Check BP, urine (output & any protein?), blood results; check presentations; IV access; bloods; synto in the room; review CTG and progress	+	You (after Rooms 1 and 2) and the SHO; AK to report to you on observations, do (or chase up) bloods, gain IV access; and prepare synto
5	Dillon	History; abdo/pelvic exam; FH (or CTG); MSU; vaginal swabs; ? fibronectin test; ? FBC	+	SHO
6	Vinci	Review of the history, CTG and progress	++	SL to do and report back to you on the CTG and VE
7	Said	Needs suturing; risk of PPH – needs assessment and preventive measures (synt, IV access; bloods)	+	DE to change roles with another m/w who can suture. m/w to report to you on assessment
8	Patel	Check BP, urine protein, I/O chart, bloods, listen to chest; examine abdomen; review/ consider antihypertensive and MgSO4; repeat bloods	++	Anaesthetic SpR
9	Surya	Intermittent auscultation	0	SU
10	Kuku	Assess – should be delivered soon. Ask m/w to commence CTG while you are reviewing Rooms 1 and 2	++	Initially m/w; if any concerns with CTG (+++) call consultant

Example 2: OSCE Q – Operating list prioritization (Prioritization, management)

Candidate's instructions

Your consultant has gone on a 2-month sabbatical. The waiting list manager has asked you to review the operation cards for the upcoming cases, and advise her on:

1. Appropriate procedures;
2. Level of priority (urgent, soon, or routine);
3. Setting (outpatient department, daycase or inpatient department);
4. Any special issues.

Note: your hospital has a new outpatient hysteroscopy unit.

You will be expected to justify your decisions.

You may make notes on the sheet and take it with you to the next station, where you will have an opportunity to discuss your decisions with the examiner.

Marks will be awarded for:

Your ability to decide on the management and prioritize the cases.

TABLE 9.3

Name	Age	Details	Procedures and work-up	Priority	Setting	Special issues/comments
Gower	32	32-w size fibroid uterus; menorrhagia; HB 7; Jehovah's Witness; two children – family complete				
Akrem	58	PMB; USS-ET = 3 mm; MI at the age of 52; unstable angina and diabetes (type 1)				
Warne	32	8/12 postnatal-breastfeeding; booked for refashioning of episiotomy scar (severe dyspareunia)				
Khan	36	Wants to be sterilized; 120 kg; X2 LSCS; laparotomy for peritonitis following appendicitis; two children; three TOPs; doesn't want 'unnatural hormones' including Depo, implants and Mirena				
Hussain	24	Subfertility for 3 years; booked for lap & dye; no previous history of pelvic pathology or PID				
Lara	23	Severe dyskaryosis; punch biopsy = CIN III; carer for a child with learning difficulties				
Mendis	68	Procedentia, treated with shelf pessary; mild angina; recent new relationship – wish to have sex (and therefore shelf pessary removed)				
Tunga	35	8-months history of cyclical pelvic pain; empirical treatment for endometriosis – no improvements in symptoms. Doesn't speak English				
Gatting	24	Recurrent miscarriages; booked for a hysteroscopy for assessment for uterine cavity abnormalities				
Gooch	64	Vulval cancer; discussed in MDT meeting; for vulvectomy				

Examiner's instructions

Candidates have 14 minutes to:

- Demonstrate their ability to decide on appropriate management.
- Demonstrate their ability to prioritize cases appropriately.

Marks should be awarded according to the structured mark sheet provided.

Structured mark sheet and model answers

Gower	0	1	2	3	4
Akrem	0	1	2	3	4
Warne	0	1	2	3	4
Khan	0	1	2	3	4
Hussain	0	1	2	3	4
Lara	0	1	2	3	4
Mendis	0	1	2	3	4
Tunga	0	1	2	3	4
Gatting	0	1	2	3	4
Gooch	0	1	2	3	4

Gross mark: $/40 \times \frac{1}{2}$

Total: **/20**

TABLE 9.4

Name	Age	Details	Procedures and work-up	Priority	Setting	Special issues/comments
Gower	32	32-w size fiboid uterus; monorrhagia; HB 7; Jehovah's Witness; 2 children – family complete	FeSO4, GnRH analogues; once Hb improved, TAH or SAH [? erythropoietin; ? blood salvage and autotransfusion]	Soon (but only after Hb improved)	Inpatient	Consent and counselling
Akrem	58	PMB; USS-ET = 3 mm; MI at the age of 52; unstable angina and diabetes (type 1)	OPD hysteroscopy and biopsy	Urgent	OPD	High risk for anaesthesia; thin ET reassuring
Warne	32	8/12 postnatal-breastfeeding; booked for refashioning of episiotomy scar (severe dyspareunia)	Fenton's procedure	Urgent	Daycase	Childcare?; First case on the list; if needs to be inpatient, side room to aid breastfeeding
Khan	36	Wants to be sterilized; 120 kg; X2 LSCS; laparotomy for peritonitis following appendicitis; 2 children; 3 TOPs; doesn't want 'unnatural hormones' including Depo, implants and Mirena	Consider vasectomy or Essure; ensure not pregnant on the day of procedure	Routine	OPD	High operative and anaesthetic risk – best to avoid laparoscopic sterilization
Hussain	24	Subfertility for 3 years; booked for lap & dye; no previous history of pelvic pathology or PID	Consider HSG or HyCoSy (as per RCOG guidelines)	Routine	OPD/ daycase	Ensure semen analysis done and ovulation confirmed before tubal assessment
Lara	23	Severe dyskaryosis; punch biopsy = CIN III; carer for a child with learning difficulties	Needs LLETZ	Urgent	OPD/ daycase	Early notice to make arrangements for the child
Mendis	68	Procedentia, treated with shelf pessary; mild angina; recent new relationship – wish to have sex (and therefore shelf pessary removed)	Vaginal hysterectomy± repair; needs preop bloods, ECG, CXR and anaesthetic review (± write to cardiologist for info)	Routine	Inpatient	Help at home?
Tunga	35	8-months history of cyclical pelvic pain; empirical treatment for endometriosis – no improvements in symptoms. Doesn't speak English	Diagnostic laparoscopy	Routine	Daycase	Translator needed for consenting

TABLE 9.4 *(continued)*

Name	Age	Details	Procedures and work-up	Priority	Setting	Special issues/comments
Gatting	24	Recurrent miscarriages; booked for a hysteroscopy for assessment for uterine cavity abnormalities	High resolution USS or HyCoSy cavity, check more appropriate	Routine	OPD	Ensure other investigations completed, e.g. APS, karyotype
Gooch	64	Vulval cancer; discussed in MDT meeting; for vulvectomy	Radical vulvectomy and lymphadenectomy (by gynaeoncologist)	Urgent	Inpatient	Ensure preop work-up all done; ? chemo/ radiotherapy

Section 3

Section 3

Practice OSCE circuits

10

The OSCE Circuit

Format

The OSCE circuit lasts for 3 hours and consists of 12 varied 'stations' of 15 minutes' duration each. The bell will sound 1 minute before the conclusion of a station (i.e. at 14 minutes) to allow 1 minute for the examiner to complete the mark sheet; this is your signal to move to the next station and begin to read the relevant information.

Stations you will encounter include:

- History taking and management;
- Counselling and breaking bad news;
- Results/data interpretation;
- Critical appraisal;
- Equipment/surgery and practical techniques;
- Emergencies;
- Structured oral examinations ('vivas');
- Clinical prioritization.

Life in an exam circuit

The bell rings!

As soon as the bell rings you will be moving to your allocated station if this is the start of the exam, or if you have already started the exam, you will be moving on to the next station. The first minute allocated to each station is a

decisive minute – it often sets you up to succeed or fail that station. Thus it is important to make the best use of this minute.

The 1 minute!

The examiner gets 1 minute to mark the previous candidate. You are expected not to enter the cubicle during this minute. Instead, there are three vital tasks to be done in that minute:

- Read the question (pinned up on a board outside the cubicle);
- Understand the question;
- Start preparing the answer for the question.

Questions are generally duplicated on the board outside the cubicle and at the desk in the cubicle. Although you can read, understand and prepare the answer for the question while you are in the cubicle, it makes a great deal of sense to do these steps before you enter the cubicle. Outside the cubicle, there is no examiner or role player, and without their curious eyes on you, you are much more likely to accomplish the three vital tasks to a high quality. If you need more than 1 minute to do these tasks, *take* the extra time! It is your time; we do not need to remind you that you paid the College handsomely to purchase this time! There is absolutely no point rushing into the cubicle when you are not ready. For instance, if your previous station shook you, take the extra time to compose yourself (in addition to performing the above three vital tasks) before walking into the next cubicle. You are in control of this time – your use or misuse of it will largely determine how well you do in that particular station.

Inside an exam cubicle

Here is the moment you have been waiting for: the beginning of the end of the MRCOG exam! The moment to prove yourself! Having read, understood and prepared in your mind the answer to the question in the preceding 1 minute, you will now stride purposefully to your chair in the cubicle (without knocking down any objects on the way).

You will often find your time inside an exam cubicle to be long and noisy, but ultimately easy. The scenarios are almost always drawn from your daily practice, and thus you should be familiar with them. Here is our guide to your survival in the cubicle:

- 'Be yourself' – this is admittedly easier said than done, but it is important not to become too excited or too animated to impress the examiner. Remember you want to come across as confident, calm and competent.

- Talk slowly and purposefully. By talking 'slowly' we do not mean that you should stretch out every word; however, most of us have a tendency to talk fast, especially when a little stressed, and if we slow down marginally, it does wonders to the effectiveness of our communication. Practise this.
- Make good eye contact! Do not look at the instruction sheet too often.
- Use non-medical language with role players (see section 3.3).
- Listen to the role player – do not interrupt too much (however, be in charge; see Chapter 3).
- Invite questions.
- Always show that you are a 'safe' doctor.

Frequently asked questions

Should I greet the examiner (in a role player station)?

It is always polite to greet another person, especially if you are going to be sharing a small cubicle with that person for 14 minutes. A quick 'Hello' and handshake to the examiner, and your natural full greeting to the role player: *'Good Morning Mrs Taylor! I am Dr Smith'* is the right approach. The advice to 'ignore the examiner' relates to the fact that you should not be engaging the examiner once you have started the consultation with the role player. Greeting both the examiner and the role player at the outset, however, is a polite gesture and likely to generate a good impression of you.

Should I shake hands?

Do if this is what you normally do. We recommend this, based on evidence (see Chapter 3). However, if this does not come naturally to you, or you wish to avoid this for personal or other reasons, then it is acceptable not to offer your hand.

Should I make notes during the consultation?

The only purpose of any notes you make is to aid you. Remember, you will not be marked on your notes and no medicolegal expert will be going through your notes as can potentially happen with notes that you make in daily practice. Therefore, brief 'bullet point' notes to help you is all that is required.

If the examiner is quiet in the exam, is that a bad sign?

If the examiner is quiet and does not appear to agree or disagree with what you say (e.g. in an audit station), they are likely to have been instructed to do so (to ensure they do not advantage or disadvantage any candidates). Moreover, if the role player looks angry, bored or irritated with you, again she is likely to have been instructed to be so. So, do not take it personally and do not get flustered (see Chapter 3 for advice on how to deal with difficult situations).

What are my chances if I completely mess up a station?

Remind yourself you still have nine other stations in which to prove yourself. It is perfectly possible to pass the exam even if you completely mess up one station or even two. Take time to compose yourself (see above). It will be detrimental to carry any negative 'baggage' from one station to the next.

You should never 'completely mess up a station' if you have a fall-back strategy. For instance, you may be faced with counselling a woman with vaginal cancer. Even with little knowledge of this topic, you can still provide the patient with sensitive and empathetic care (see Chapter 3) and address general issues [e.g. *'We will need to ascertain the extent of the cancer (staging)'* and *'A team of experts including doctors, nurses and counsellors will be caring for you (multidisciplinary care in a cancer centre)'*]. You can then agree to get back with more specific information [*'I will arrange for a discussion of the details amongst experts (multidisciplinary team meeting), and will then be sure to get back to you with exact details on treatment'*]. So, although you may have known very little about vaginal cancer, you will have scored several marks.

What if I do not understand the question?

There are two distinct scenarios:

1. You haven't *heard* the question (because the examiner or role player spoke softly or the exam hall was noisy);
2. You have not *understood* the question.

For the former, you will need to say: *'I am sorry; I didn't hear the question very well. Could you please repeat it for me?'* For the latter, you will need to say: *'I am sorry; I am unable to understand the question; could you please rephrase it for me?'*

If you have not understood the question and you ask the examiner to repeat it, they will do just that, and you will still be none the wiser. Thus it is important to use the words 'repeat' and 'rephrase' correctly.

Answer the question: A common mistake to avoid

If the question is 'what would you do?', tell the examiner what *you* would do, and not 'there are two schools of thought ...' or 'RCOG guideline states ...' The examiner is seeking your views, taking you to be an independent and competent practitioner who is able to provide your own distilled thoughts on the question; reciting the thoughts of others is unlikely to be helpful. So, it is important to start the answer with, *'In this situation, I would ...'*. Once you have said what *you* would do, then it would be reasonable to contextualize your actions, e.g. by stating the RCOG guidelines and explaining any variance.

Top tip: Set the agenda

Communicate the aim/objectives/purpose of the consultation/question at the beginning, and check this is what the role player or examiner also has in mind! This is not just for the exam, but a useful habit in almost every clinical encounter. Managers call this 'setting the agenda'. This step often differentiates the professionals from the amateurs amongst you.

Example 1
'Mrs Smith, I have a copy of the letter from your doctor, which tells me you have heavy periods. What I would like to do is to find out more about this and any other problems, examine you, arrange some investigations, and then discuss the treatment possibilities. Is this OK with you?'

Example 2
'I have been asked to develop an audit to assess steroid use in women with threatened preterm labour. I will do this by (a) defining the criteria and standard for good practice; (b) collecting data on current practice; (c) analyzing the data; (d) presenting the results to the relevant stakeholders; (e) making necessary changes to practice, and finally (f) closing the audit loop, by re-auditing to see if the changes implemented have had the desired effect. I will now provide details on each of these steps ...'

11

Practice circuit 1

- Duration – 3 hours
- Structure – 12 stations × 15 minutes
- Additional information: The bell will sound 1 minute before the conclusion of the station (i.e. at 14 minutes) to allow 1 minute for the examiner to complete the mark sheet and during which time you will move to the next station and begin to read the relevant information.

In addition to questions, detailed structured mark sheets and case notes are provided.

Station 1 – Gynaecology on-call (preparatory station)

Candidate's instructions

You are the SpR on-call for gynaecology. It is 5 pm and the following on-call problems have been handed over to you:

1. *Patient 1*: A 54-year-old diabetic woman who is day 3 post-hysterectomy complaining of increasingly severe chest pain and shortness of breath for the last 20 minutes.
2. *Patient 2*: A 66-year-old woman complaining of severe discomfort because she has been unable to pass urine all day since removal of her urinary catheter this morning following an anterior vaginal repair.
3. *Patient 3*: A 22-year-old woman just admitted with heavy vaginal bleeding at 10 weeks' gestation. The nurse informs you that she is pale, clammy with a heart rate of 100 and a blood pressure of 90/60.

4. *Patient 4*: A 34-year-old woman with a confirmed tubal ectopic pregnancy on scan who is consented and awaiting theatre. She has been asymptomatic but is now complaining of severe abdominal pain and breathlessness.
5. *Patient 5*: A 72-year-old woman who has passed 50 ml over the last 6 hours since returning from theatre for a staging laparotomy for ovarian cancer.
6. *Patient 6*: The general surgeons want an urgent opinion in the emergency operating theatre on a 26-year-old woman on whom they have performed a laparotomy for a presumed appendicitis, but have found an inflamed pelvis full of pus and an ovarian mass.
7. *Patient 7*: A family who have been waiting for the last 3 hours for someone from the medical staff to come and discuss with them today's laparoscopy findings on their 17-year-old daughter. They are extremely angry about the delay and are shouting at the nursing staff.

The staff available to you in hospital are:

- One GP SHO;
- One charge nurse;
- Three trained (staff grade) nurses ('A', 'B', 'C');
- One healthcare assistant (HCA) (untrained nursing auxiliary);
- Two on-call anaesthetic SpRs (first and second on);
- O&G consultant on-call is at home.

Your task is to prioritize and manage the emergency cases. You have 15 minutes preparation time.

Marks will be awarded for:

- Ability to prioritize emergency cases;
- Ability to delegate appropriately emergency work;
- Ability to manage emergency cases.

Station 2 – Gynaecology on-call (Prioritization, management)

Your task is to prioritize and manage the emergency cases.

Structured mark sheet

Identification of management tasks, prioritization and delegation.

Patient 1: **A 54-year-old diabetic woman who is day 3 post-hysterectomy complaining of increasingly severe chest pain and shortness of breath for the last 20 minutes.**

- **Management**: This patient needs thorough medical assessment to exclude serious pathology, e.g. PE, MI, RTI. Will need history/examination, vital signs, O_2 saturations $\pm$ ABGs, ECG, CXR, FBC, U&Es.
- **Staff**: SHO + trained nurse A.
- **Priority**: High (immediate attention).

Patient 2: **A 66-year-old woman complaining of severe discomfort because she has been unable to pass urine all day since removal of her urinary catheter this morning following an anterior vaginal repair.**

- **Management**: This patient needs urinary catheterization.
- **Staff**: Trained nurse B.
- **Priority**: Medium (pressing attention).

Patient 3: **A 22-year-old woman just admitted with heavy vaginal bleeding at 10 weeks' gestation. The nurse informs you that she is pale, clammy with a heart rate of 100 and a blood pressure of 90/60.**

- **Management**: This patient needs thorough gynaecological assessment and resuscitation – this is a threatened miscarriage associated with haemodynamic shock. She requires resuscitation ('ABCs' – O_2, IV access, fluids, FBC $\pm$ clotting, G&S/cross-match, U&Es) and pelvic examination to check cervical os for inevitable miscarriage/products of conception/blood clot within the cervical canal producing a vaso-vagal response (removal will probably help resolve situation) or, if shock due to acute haemorrhage, requires administration of uterotonic agents, blood transfusion, cross-match and preparation for emergency theatre (call on-call anaesthetist).
- **Staff** – You (SpR), trained nurse C $\pm$ second on anaesthetic SpR.
- **Priority** – High (immediate attention).

Patient 4: **A 34-year-old woman with a confirmed tubal ectopic pregnancy on scan who is consented and awaiting theatre. She has been asymptomatic but is now complaining of severe abdominal pain and breathlessness.**

- **Management**: This patient needs thorough gynaecological assessment to exclude ruptures/leaking ectopic pregnancy. History (shoulder tip pain), vital signs (tachycardia, hypotension), abdominal examination (not vaginal) to diagnose peritonitis (rigidity, acute tenderness), transabdominal USS (if accredited) to look for echogenic free fluid suggestive of blood. If ruptured ectopic diagnosed then check Hb, arrange cross-match 4 units and summon the second-on anaesthetist and consultant on-call from home.
- **Staff** – You (SpR), charge nurse, consultant on-call from home to attend ± second on anaesthetic SpR.
- **Priority** – High (immediate attention).

Patient 5: **A 72-year-old woman who has passed 50 ml over the last 6 hours since returning from theatre for a staging laparotomy for ovarian cancer.**

- **Management**: This patient needs thorough medical/gynaecological assessment to diagnose cause of oliguria (i.e. pre-renal, renal, post-renal impairment). Needs quick history (any renal/cardiac problems), input/output (fluid balance assessed), theatre notes (EBL), vital signs, general exam (cardiogenic, fluid overload, pulmonary oedema, etc), abdominal/pelvic exam (postoperative haemorrhage). Check catheter not occluded/incorrectly sited, blocked, FBC, U&E, Cr, profile (± ECG/CXR) ± on-call RMO for medical review.
- **Staff**: SHO, trained nurse.
- **Priority**: Medium (pressing attention).

Patient 6: **The general surgeons want an urgent opinion in the emergency operating theatre on a 26-year-old woman on whom they have performed a laparotomy for a presumed appendicitis, but have found an inflamed pelvis full of pus and an ovarian mass.**

- **Management** – Ask charge nurse to call consultant on-call to attend and contact theatre to expect delay.
- **Staff** – consultant to attend.
- **Priority** – medium (pressing attention).

Patient 7: **A family who have been waiting for the last 3 hours for someone from the medical staff to come and discuss with them today's laparoscopy findings on their 17-year-old daughter. They are extremely angry about the delay and are shouting at the nursing staff.**

- **Management** – Ask HCA to speak to the family, convey apologies and workload on the department. Take the family off the ward to an appropriate sitting area and offer to come back with refreshments. Call hospital porters/security to remove the relatives if they continue to be disruptive.
- **Staff** – HCA.
- **Priority** – Low (clinically), but urgent non-clinical attention to prevent compromise of other patient care.

Management [8]

0   1   2   3   4   5   6   7   8

Prioritization and delegation [8]

0   1   2   3   4   5   6   7   8

Global score [4]

0   1   2   3   4

Total: /20

Case notes

These clinical scenarios are an opportunity to shine and display your clinical acumen and experience ('break free of the confines of theoretical knowledge'). Adopt a logical, calm and considered approach. Just think about what you would actually do faced with such a busy situation on-call.

Clinical situations are rarely 'cut and dry' and much of the delegation and subsequent responses will depend upon the dynamic clinical situation (results of assessments, investigations, changes in clinical state), so slight variation from the standardized 'examiner's mark sheet' is acceptable as long as the main priorities are identified and acted upon.

It is clear from the scenarios given here that the problems in the department require consultant presence due to the workload ('extra pair of hands') and potential seriousness (need consultant-level experience) of some of the problems. This should be recognized immediately and the consultant should be summoned by the charge nurse (whilst you delegate tasks).

Patients 1, 3 and 4 are the top priorities as they are all acute, potentially life-threatening emergencies. Patients 3 and 4 require gynaecological expertise immediately. In such a situation, quick assessments and rational action is of paramount importance. Once assessments are made, further tasks (booking theatre, arranging bloods, fluids) can then be delegated, but you need to be aware of the problems that only you have the necessary skills to deal with.

Patient 5 is the patient likely to keep you up all night. Although she is a priority as she may deteriorate rapidly (clinical problems in the elderly can often be underestimated), in the busy situation painted here she will have to wait.

Acute urinary retention is extremely painful and is a situation that can be quickly rectified, so one of your trained nurses should be deployed to catheterize Patient 2, and then make themselves available to aid the clinical care of patients 1, 3, 4 and 5.

Station 3 – Birth trauma and anger (Communication, counselling)

Candidate's instructions

You are about so see Sheila Shaw, a 34-year-old accountant. You delivered her first baby 3 days ago and the baby is on the special care baby unit as a precaution because of feeding difficulties and jaundice. She had an emergency caesarean section at full dilatation for a deep transverse arrest after a failed trial of forceps delivery. The baby had some bruising arising from your forceps delivery and has a 3 cm laceration over the right cheek where you inadvertently cut him during the caesarean section.

You are about to see Sheila on the ward. The midwives have told you that she is very angry about what has happened.

Your task is to explain what has happened and to handle the patient's concerns.

Marks will be awarded for:

- Ability to deal appropriately with a difficult situation;
- Ability to counsel an angry patient.

Role player's instructions

At this station you are very angry and upset.

You are Sheila Shaw, a 34-year-old accountant, and have just had your first baby 3 days ago. You and your partner have found the whole experience deeply traumatic.

You had an emergency caesarean section under general anaesthetic (i.e. you were put to sleep). You delivered a baby boy, Thomas. The whole experience was a blur and you do not feel you were adequately informed about what was about to happen to you. You expected to have the delivery under an 'epidural' (i.e. a regional anaesthetic, so you would be awake during the delivery).

When you woke up you were told that Thomas was on the special care baby unit. Your husband saw Thomas and he had a 'cut' on his face, which was covered with 'steri-strips' (sticky tapes to hold the wound together). Your son looked 'bruised and swollen' with obvious forceps marks over his skull and eyes.

The neonatal unit nurses have told you that Thomas is not feeding well because he is in pain from his 'traumatic delivery' and the bruising that it caused has led to his jaundice and the need for phototherapy (blue light therapy used to treat the jaundice).

You expected child birth to be a happy, enriching experience but instead you and your husband feel traumatized. You wanted to have more children, but have found the whole experience so awful that you do not feel you can go through any further pregnancies.

You blame this doctor for the way you feel and for the problems your baby has had. You want the doctor to explain why they cut and bruised your baby and what they think about the standard of care you received.

Questions/remarks you should ask/make during the consultation are:

1. No-one explained what was going to happen to me or my husband, which left us feeling very frightened.
2. Why did you cut my baby during a routine caesarean section? Surely you are incompetent?
3. My baby's face is bruised and swollen because of the attempted forceps delivery that you performed. Why weren't you more careful?
4. Is my baby going to be 'brain damaged'?
5. I want to make a formal complaint and sue the hospital for their poor care.

Examiner's instructions

The candidate has 14 minutes to demonstrate the following:

- Ability to deal appropriately with a difficult situation.
- Ability to communicate and counsel an angry patient.
- Ability to deal adequately with the patient's concerns.

Structured mark sheet

Communication/counselling skills [8]

- Introduction:
  - Greet, introduce, gain permission, eye contact;
  - Sympathetic approach – not responding aggressively;
  - Respectfully use the patient's name in your reply. When a person is very angry, using her name in a respectful way can ease the situation – do not be over familiar – 'Sheila' is inappropriate.
- Approach:
  - Speak in a calm, quiet manner;
  - Listen attentively – do not interrupt. Let the patient speak her mind without interruption. Encourage her to disclose her feelings, worries and concerns;
  - Use supportive non-verbal communication such as nodding, looks of concern, maintaining eye contact;
  - Defuse anger – do *not* counter it with your own anger or ignore it; this will be counterproductive;
  - Need to address/acknowledge/validate the emotion, e.g. *'This must be difficult for you. Can you tell me how you are feeling?' 'You seem very angry?'*, or even acknowledge her right to be angry, *'I can see that you are angry, and I think I would be too in this situation'*.
  - Display empathy and concern; this can help the patient feel understood. Paraphrasing the patient's comments is an effective way to convey that you have listened and are seeking to understand: *'So you feel very annoyed that no-one explained the situation to you ....' 'I can see how angry you are about what happened ...'*, *'It must be hard for you with your baby on the special care unit ...'*.

0   1   2   3   4   5   6   7   8

Dealing with questions/concerns [8]

- Apologies and context:
  - Apologize for the apparent lack of effective communication. *'I'm sorry if we failed to explain things to you adequately'* or *'I'm sorry if you feel we let you down/did not perform as we would have liked to.'* Context – *'LW can be very busy,' 'We were trying to do our best for you and your baby'*. Finish off with an apology again, but avoid 'over rationalizing'. The main aim is to deal with the patient's feelings/emotions. Logic should take a back seat;
  - Apologize for birth trauma – as above. Context – *'Bruising following forceps deliveries is not uncommon and usually quickly resolves, but I'm sorry this may have made his jaundice worse'*;
  - The cut face definitely deserves an apology and a show of insight into the concern it has caused – best just to express how sorry you are that this has happened: *'I always aim to be very gentle and careful when surgically delivering babies, so I am extremely disappointed and sorry about what has happened'*;
  - Reassure that although you are sorry that the baby is externally bruised and has a laceration, and is requiring treatment for jaundice and help with feeding, the paediatricians are not worried about serious neurological injury.
- Explain access to complaints procedures, e.g. PALS, be helpful, do not appear defensive. Do not become upset or anxious about the threat to sue.
- Round up, summarize and offer to meet again with partner to answer further questions/concerns if necessary: *'Please don't hesitate to contact me via …'.*

0   1   2   3   4   5   6   7   8

Global score

0   1   2   3   4

Total: **/20**

Case notes

When dealing with an angry patient or relative, whether rational or irrational, you should aim to resolve conflict positively. You will know when you have been successful because you will feel that you handled the situation in a professional, dignified manner. Some tips to help achieve this are:

- Environment – move the patient to a quiet area (the angry patient with an audience will be less likely to accept your point of view).
- Respectfully use the patient's name in your reply. When a person is very angry, using her name in a respectful way can ease the situation.

- Listen – let the patient speak her mind without interruption.
- Display empathy and concern – this can help the patient feel she is understood. Paraphrasing the patient's comments is an effective way to convey that you have listened and are seeking to understand. *'So you feel like it's so unfair that the cancer appeared out of nowhere after all these years.'*
- Avoid rationalizing – put yourself in the patient's shoes for just a moment and consider whether your rationalization is an explanation or an excuse. It is tempting, when faced with an angry individual, to explain the situation in such a way as to imply that the anger is inappropriate. In fact, when emotions are involved, logic has no place and it is best to work with feelings. Indeed it is important to encourage expression of feelings: *'Can you tell me how you are feeling'.*
- Acknowledge the emotion – *'You seem to be very angry?'* It is crucial to validate feelings so the angry person feels that you are listening. Attempting to defuse the anger, countering it with your own anger or ignoring it will be counterproductive. Acknowledging the patient's right to be angry will help start the healing process and solidify the therapeutic relationship.
- Acknowledge the anger and demonstrate your understanding: *'I can see how angry you are about what happened ...'*, *'It must be hard for you with your baby on the special care unit ...'*; be sincere: *'I understand how you feel ...'.*

Station 4 – Operative vaginal delivery: forceps (Practical competencies)

Candidate's instructions

At this station you will have 14 minutes to answer questions and demonstrate practical competencies in relation to operative vaginal delivery.

The examiner will ask you a series of questions about the practice of operative vaginal delivery and will provide you with relevant instruments as part of the structured viva.

Marks will be awarded for:

- Your ability to answer the questions about indications and techniques of operative vaginal delivery;
- Your appreciation and understanding of safety issues;
- Your knowledge and application of instrumentation.

Examiner's instructions

This is a structured viva and assessment of practical skills. At this station, the candidate has 14 minutes to answer questions related to endoscopic surgery and to demonstrate the relevant competencies.

You should ask the candidate the questions on your mark sheet and provide the candidate with the obstetric forceps and pelvic/fetal model as appropriate. You can prompt the candidate if necessary, but this requirement should be reflected in the marks awarded.

You should have the following equipment:

- Kielland's forceps;
- Simpson's or Neville Barnes' forceps;
- Pelvic model;
- 'Fetal' doll.

Questions to be asked:

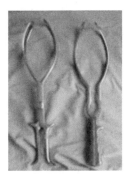

Give the candidate the Kielland's forceps.
1. Ask the candidate to identify this instrument, give the indication for its use and describe the key features facilitating its use (mid-cavity rotation).

Give the candidate the non-rotational 'classic' mid-cavity forceps (Simpson's).
2. Ask the candidate to identify this instrument and give the indications for its use.
3. Assuming you are a skilled, trained operator, what clinical criteria need to be satisfied prior to their routine use?

Give the candidate the Simpson's forceps and hold the model of the female pelvis and baby.
4. Ask the candidate to show and describe how they would conduct a non-rotational forceps delivery.

Structured mark sheet

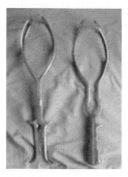

1. Ask the candidate to identify this instrument, give the indication for its use and describe the key features facilitating its use (mid-cavity rotation). [1]

- Kielland's rotational forceps.
- Rotational delivery (correct OP or OT positions).
- Sliding lock, cephalic curve but no (minimal) pelvic curve.

0   1

2. Ask the candidate to identify the instrument and give the indications for its use? [4]

- Non-rotational forceps.
- Indications:
  - Fetal – presumed fetal compromise;
  - Maternal – medical indications to avoid Valsalva (e.g. cardiac disease, Class III or IVa hypertensive crises, cerebral vascular disease, particularly uncorrected cerebral vascular malformations, myasthenia gravis, spinal cord injury);
  - Inadequate progress: (1) nulliparous women: lack of continuing progress for 3 hours (total of active and passive second stage labour) progress with regional anaesthesia, or 2 hours without regional anaesthesia; (2) multiparous women: lack of continuing progress for 2 hours (total of active and passive second stage labour) with regional anaesthesia, or 1 hour without regional anaesthesia; (3) maternal fatigue/exhaustion.

0   1   2   3   4

3. Assuming you are a skilled, trained operator, what clinical criteria need to be satisfied prior to their routine use? **[5]**

- Head is ≤ 1/5 palpable per abdomen.
- Cervix is fully dilated.
- Membranes ruptured.
- Maternal bladder has been emptied recently (indwelling catheter should be removed or balloon deflated).
- Vertex presentation.
- OA < 45° from direct (midline) position or low direct OP (station +2).
- Full engagement of the head (not above ischial spines, i.e. > 0 station, *but* take account of abdominal examination also).
- Exact position of the head determined (and pelvis is considered adequate).
- Appropriate analgesia – regional or pudendal block.
- Informed maternal consent (clear explanation given) and cooperation.
- Good uterine contractions.

0   1   2   3   4   5

4. Ask the candidate to show and describe how they would conduct a non-rotational forceps delivery **[6]**

- Position patient in lithotomy position.
- Check the forceps – 'dry run', put them together to check they are a 'pair' and 'true' (i.e. fit together, ≥ 9 cm between two blades).
- Apply lubricant (e.g. Hibitane cream).
- Atraumatic application of blades:
  - Warn patient;
  - Await uterine relaxation (abandon if uterine contraction intervenes);
  - Gentle, wide sweep at correct angle (in line with opposite inguinal ligament);
  - Vaginal hand to guide and protect vagina/baby (use this hand to rotate/stabilize head in the DOA position if LOA/LOP (< 45°) position;
  - Easy locking of blades – remove and replace if resistance.
- Relax locking whilst awaiting contraction. Vaginal examination to check correct application position – sagittal suture palpable in the midline (DOA/DOP).
- Gentle traction beginning with the peak of each contraction/maternal effort (midwife and/or you coach the mother) in the plane of the pelvis (pelvic axis) for the duration of the contraction.
- Make an episiotomy when there is sufficient descent such that delivery is imminent (usually as the vertex reaches the vaginal outlet (reaches pelvic

floor/perineum). Occasionally required sooner if bleeding following blade application (avoid spiral tears) or more room required to apply blades.

- As the head crowns, change the angle of traction through 90° and control delivery of head [protect perineum with hand, mother to stop pushing ('pant')].
- Check neck for cord – loosen, take off neck and deliver shoulders with next contraction/maternal effort after restitution with external rotation and lateral flexion. Deliver placenta (active third stage ± elective oxytocin infusion – risk PPH).
- Careful vaginal/perineal/rectal examination and repair episiotomy/tears (check baby's head for significant bruising, confirm correct blade application, explain to parents bruising is to be expected – should resolve in 7 days).
- Documentation (and review prior to discharge).

0   1   2   3   4   5   6

Global score   **[4]**

0   1   2   3   4

Total: **/20**

Case notes

Before the exam, spend an hour reading a basic (undergraduate will do) obstetric textbook to mug up on definitions, e.g. lie, presentation, position, vertex, engagement, mechanism of normal labour and basic pelvic anatomy (inlet, mid-cavity, outlet, pelvic conjugate), so that an examiner does not catch you out. You should, however, be confident at demonstrating the practical side of instrumental delivery as you do it on-call every day! Next time you conduct such a delivery aim to do it in a 'textbook' fashion, thinking about each step you take, including communication with the mother.

Of all deliveries, 10–15% are operative vaginal deliveries. As with any surgical intervention, adverse events are possible and, in the case of a baby, the consequences can be catastrophic if instrumental delivery is badly executed. To reduce potential morbidity for both the mother and the baby requires good examination skills, an awareness of prerequisites for instrumental delivery, good technique and, above all, sound clinical judgement (particularly when to abandon procedures and revert to caesarean section). It is therefore important that you convey to the examiner the priority of safety considerations and come across as a mature, competent and safe clinician.

Operative deliveries on the labour ward (including caesarean section) are a good topic to set an audit question on. It is thus, in addition to clinical practice, worth thinking about how you would audit important outcomes in operative deliveries in obstetrics (rates, complications, documentation, training, complaints, medicolegal issues).

Further reading

Johanson RB. 2003: Ventouse and forceps delivery: In: Johanson R, Cox C, Grady K, Howell C, eds. *Managing Obstetric Emergencies and Trauma.* The MOET Course Manual. London: RCOG Press: Chapter 24.

RCOG Green Top Guideline. Operative Vaginal Delivery (26) – 2005 (available at: www.rcog.org.uk/index.asp?PageID=523).

Station 5 – Third-degree tears (Preparatory station)

Candidate's instructions

The consultant you work for is head of clinical risk management in the hospital obstetric department. He has been informed by the hospital legal department that litigation is proceeding in two cases of unrecognized third-degree tears, leading to one case of symptomatic recto-vaginal septum and another of intractable faecal urgency and incontinence necessitating a colostomy prior to a secondary repair. Both cases involved the use of obstetric forceps by obstetricians in training grades.

He has approached you as his SpR to conduct an audit into third-degree tears and from this to make recommendations with the aim of improving the quality of care provided and reducing future risks of litigation.

You have 15 minutes to decide how you would design and conduct this audit and discuss this with the examiner. The examiner will then give you the findings of your audit and ask you to make recommendations in light of these findings.

Marks will be awarded for:

- Designing an appropriate audit;
- Explaining how you would conduct the audit;
- Making appropriate inferences from the results to enable appropriate recommendations to be made.

Station 6 – Third-degree tears (Audit, risk management)

Candidate's instructions

Discuss with the examiner how you would design and conduct this audit. The examiner will then give you the findings of your audit and ask you to make recommendations in light of these findings.

Marks will be awarded for:

- Designing an appropriate audit;
- Explaining how you would conduct the audit;
- Making appropriate inferences from the results to enable the making of appropriate recommendations.

Examiner's instructions

Candidates need to cover the areas of discussion on the structured mark sheet and can be prompted by a specific question if they do not mention them spontaneously.

Once the candidate has outlined how they will design and conduct an appropriate audit, then give them the following results of the audit and ask them to make some appropriate recommendations in light of this information.

1. The incidence of third-/fourth-degree tears is 12% of all instrumental deliveries.
2. No uniform definition or documentation of anal trauma is documented in the case notes.
3. 80% of all repairs were conducted by junior SpRs (year 1–3) or SHOs.
4. Braided polyglactin (Vicryl™) was used to repair the anal sphincter in all cases.
5. 50% of repairs were performed in the delivery room.
6. Broad-spectrum antibiotics were administered in 40% of cases.
7. Laxatives were prescribed in 60% of cases.
8. Adequate documentation of the injury and follow-up plan was documented explicitly in 10% of cases prior to hospital discharge.
9. Follow-up in outpatients following anal trauma occurred in 10% of cases, although this varied according to consultant.

Structured mark sheet

Design [6]

- Establish clear aims and objectives (focus audit to concerns expressed in the first instance):
  - Establish incidence of third-degree tears (perineal/anal trauma) and associated risk factors (in this audit, the risk factors to assess are operative vaginal delivery and grade of obstetrician);
  - Establish current practice for managing third-degree tears and compare this practice against defined standards of best quality, contemporary care.
- Define quality standards. Obtain these from published guidelines, systematic reviews, primary evidence, expert opinion – ask Trust librarian to do this, present plans at appropriate forum where senior obstetricians are available or correspond mailshot/questionnaire by e-mail/post.

Quality standards for repair of third-/fourth-degree tears

1. All women having a vaginal delivery should have a systematic examination of the perineum, vagina and rectum to assess the severity of damage prior to suturing and a uniform definition of severity and degree of injury should be employed and documented in the case notes.
2. The rate of third-/fourth-degree tears following instrumental vaginal delivery should be < 10% of all such deliveries.
3. All women having instrumental delivery or who have extensive perineal injury should be examined by an experienced obstetrician, trained in the recognition and management of perineal tears.
4. All repairs should be conducted by or under the direct supervision of an experienced (e.g. year 4/5 SpR upwards) obstetrician.
5. All repairs should be carried out in an operating theatre, under regional or general anaesthesia.
6. Clearly documented in the operation notes should be: anatomical structures involved; method of repair; and suture materials – fine (e.g. 2–0, 3–0), non-absorbable [e.g. polypropylene (Prolene)] or long-acting monofilament sutures [e.g. Polydioxanone™ (PDS) should be used to repair the anal sphincter complex].
7. Broad-spectrum antibiotics (e.g. augmentin, cephalexin and metronidazole) should be used intraoperatively and in the postoperative period.
8. Laxatives should be prescribed for 7–14 days after the repair (e.g. stool softener such as Lactulose™ and a bulking agent such as Fybogel™).

Quality standards for repair of third-/fourth-degree tears
(continued)

9. All woman must be fully informed about the nature of the injury and importance of subsequent follow-up and this documented in the case notes prior to discharge from hospital.
10. All women who have had a third- or fourth-degree tear repaired should be offered a planned follow-up at 6–12 months by a gynaecologist with an interest in anorectal dysfunction or a colorectal surgeon, and rates of ongoing faecal symptoms and incontinence recorded.

- Decide how to collect data – prospective/retrospective (retrospective probably better in this case to establish current practice quicker, so enabling institution of recommendations from a risk management perspective).

0   1   2   3   4   5   6

Conduct   [6]

- Determine an adequate sample size (i.e. large enough to be assessed robustly, but of a realistic size that enables completion).
- Determine an adequate time frame, e.g. last year (i.e. long enough to be assessed robustly, but of a realistic length to enable completion).
- Design an explicit data collection form/electronic database to assess pre-specified standards.
- Collect data:
  - Liaise with management, clinical risk and IT to ascertain what data are collected routinely electronically [e.g. number of deliveries – normal or instrumental (obtain denominator)] and if complications of delivery, including third-degree tears, are coded;
  - If not coded look at delivery records on the labour ward or if not documented at all look at all instrumental deliveries;
  - Case note review will be necessary to obtain documentary evidence – liaise with the audit department/lead to help obtain medical records.
- Enter data onto database and analyze to produce usable, understandable results.
- Disseminate/present/interpret results for discussion – audit meetings, oncology meetings, 'PMB' group to include all relevant stakeholders. Publish results in hospital publications, correspondence, e-mail.

0   1   2   3   4   5   6

Recommendations [4]

- As none of the quality standards was met and the incidence of anal trauma associated with instrumental deliveries was greater than that suggested in the literature (1–9%), a complete overhaul is required.
- A standardized protocol should be developed and disseminated in line with the set quality standards.
- Familiarizing and training of the obstetric senior and junior staff with this protocol is required.
- A perineal trauma clinic should be established routinely to follow-up patients to debrief (reducing litigation), assess symptoms and adequacy of repair and comprehensively identify long-term complications.
- An appropriate senior permanent member of clinical staff should be identified to take responsibility for implementation of the protocol and continuation of the audit cycle (i.e. to collect the data prospectively).
- This person should estimate the extra resources required to implement the changes and liaise with hospital management to obtain it.

0   1   2   3   4

Global score [4]

0   1   2   3   4

Total: **/20**

Case notes

It is important in audit as in research to define explicitly the conditions, processes and outcomes to be evaluated. Various definitions have been used for anal trauma (in the UK/US), but the definitions recommended by the RCOG are:

- Second-degree tear: injury to the perineum involving perineal muscles but not the anal sphincter.
- Third-degree: injury to perineum involving the anal sphincter complex (EAS and IAS): 3a: < 50% of EAS thickness torn; 3b: > 50% of EAS thickness torn; 3c: IAS torn.
- Fourth-degree: injury to perineum involving the anal sphincter complex (EAS and IAS) and rectal mucosa.
- Anal incontinence – any involuntary loss of faeces, flatus or urge incontinence that is adversely affecting a woman's quality of life.

In many audits, as in this one, it can be impractical to obtain complete data retrospectively. In this example it would have been ideal to obtain the rates of faecal symptoms/incontinence, RV fistula, infection, breakdown of repair, etc, and to stratify these by potential prognostic factors (e.g. grade of surgeon, technique). However, such useful clinical data would be collectable in the future if a uniform follow-up pathway is used and a perineal trauma clinic established to document standard information prospectively.

The role of primary overlap repair has been overstated as the best evidence available from a randomized controlled trial did not show that the overlap method is superior to the end-to-end (approximation) method in terms of objective or subjective symptomatic outcomes. It is likely that the specifics of the method of repair are less important than recognition of the extent of the tear, and adequate suturing by an appropriately trained surgeon utilizing good technique (retrieve the retracted torn ends of the anal sphincter and bring them together without any tension), analgesia/anaesthesia, light, assistance, suture material, antibiotics, laxatives and follow-up. Regional or general anaesthesia will allow the woman to be pain-free and the anal sphincter to relax, which is essential to good repair.

From a clinical and risk management standpoint, the key message is that the occurrence of a third- or fourth-degree tear should not be considered substandard care because it is a known complication of vaginal delivery. However, failure to recognize anal sphincter damage, failure to carry out an adequate repair and failure to follow-up may be considered substandard care.

Further reading

RCOG. Understanding Audit Clinical Governance Advice No 5 (available at: www.rcog.org.uk/index.asp?PageID=476).

RCOG. Management of Third- and Fourth-Degree Perineal Tears Following Vaginal Delivery (29) – 2001 (Available at: www.rcog.org.uk/index.asp?PageID=532).

Station 7 – Premenstrual syndrome (history taking, communication, management)

Candidate's instructions

The patient you are about to see has been referred to your outpatient department by her GP.

Read the referral letter below and obtain a relevant history from the patient. Then go on to explain the diagnosis and discuss management options with her.

Dear Colleague

Re. Dawn Moore

I would be grateful if you could see this 38-year-old secretary whom I think has severe premenstrual syndrome. She complains of feeling very tearful and upset before her period is due and has recently been admitted overnight to Selly Oak Hospital following a paracetamol overdose. She is otherwise fit and well. I would be very grateful for your opinion about how to manage her condition.

Yours sincerely

Dr V Cross DRCOG MRCGP

Marks will be awarded for:

- Taking an appropriate history;
- Discussing appropriate investigation and management and demonstrating ability to communicate in a clear and empathetic manner.

Role player's instructions

You are Dawn Moore, a 38-year-old secretary. You have no gynaecological problems; your periods are regular and not painful, but you are troubled by severe emotional disturbance – uncontrollable crying, anger, low mood and irritability that tends to occur for 2 weeks before your period is due and resolves during your period. You have had these 'PMT' symptoms for many years but they have been getting worse for the last 2 years. You have tried taking evening primrose oil, which has helped your breast tenderness but not your emotional wellbeing. You are divorced with two teenage sons (delivered normally) who do not understand your change in mood and this is interfering with your relationship with them and your work colleagues and friends. Things have upset you so much that you took a paracetamol overdose recently. For 2 weeks every month you feel fine. You have been treated for depression in the past by your GP with an SSRI (paroxetine) but this was of no help. You smoke 20–30 cigarettes per day but do not drink.

Examiner's instructions

Candidates have 14 minutes to demonstrate the following:

- Ability to take an appropriate history;
- Ability to discuss appropriate investigation and management, demonstrating ability to communicate in a clear and empathetic manner.

Structured mark sheet

History [6]

- Ascertain if really PMS, i.e. what are the symptoms, are they predominantly physical (breast tenderness, abdominal bloating, headaches, constipation, dysmenorrhoea) or emotional (labile mood – irritability, tearful, depression) and when do they occur (i.e. 1–2 weeks premenstrually and disappear by the end of the period). Has she had any treatment for these symptoms; if so what and with what effect?
- Psychiatric – how serious was the suicide attempt?; has she had suicidal ideation before or since?; does she have biological symptoms of depression, any history of depression or has she seen a psychiatrist?
- General gynaecological history with particular attention to menstrual symptoms and past/future obstetric history.
- How are the symptoms affecting her quality of life (professional, emotional, social, family)?

0   1   2   3   4   5   6

Investigation [2]

- Symptom diary.
- No role for hormonal investigation.

0   1   2

Management and communication [8]

- Explanation of condition – PMS is a common symptom complex, which affects women to a varying degree and comprises both physical and emotional components. It is unclear what underlies the condition, but it has a 'hormonal' basis because the symptoms have a cyclical pattern. Functional/behavioural aspects.
- Basis for treatment – there is a range of management options available, some behavioural, some medical (many without a strong evidence base, but

may help some women – worthwhile even if placebo), some hormonal (importance of suppressing ovulation) and some surgical.

- As her symptoms are predominantly emotional – consider treatments for this:
  - Reassurance and explanation;
  - Lifestyle changes – adapt to time of month, reduce/stop smoking, aerobic exercise (proven benefit);
  - Cognitive behavioural therapy (CBT; has proven benefit but requires trained nurse/psychologist/psychiatrist);
  - Agnus castus fruit (Vitex agnus castus L extract);
  - Vitamin B_6 (pyridoxine) up to 100 mg/day;
  - Oestradiol patches + cyclical progesterone;
  - Trial of GnRH-a ± addback HRT therapy;
  - LAVH + BSO + ERT if a trial of GnRH-a ± addback HRT therapy is successful (observational evidence only).
- Not indicated in this particular case:
  - Treatments primarily for physical symptoms: diuretics for breast tenderness and bloating, NSAIDs/vitamin E for dysmenorrhoea; evening primrose oil for breast tenderness;
  - SSRIs – proven benefit but not for this case because failed treatment already (consider referral to a psychiatrist if a further SSRI or non-SSRI antidepressant is to be tried);
  - COC – unknown effectiveness and patient is a smoker.

0   1   2   3   4   5   6   7   8

Global score

0   1   2   3   4

Total: /20

Case notes

General synopsis

Premenstrual syndrome is defined as the recurrence of psychological and physical symptoms in the luteal phase, which remit in the follicular phase of the menstrual cycle.

Mild physiological symptoms occur in approximately 95% of all women of reproductive age. Approximately 5% of symptomatic women complain of such severe symptoms that their lives are completely disrupted. It is estimated that up to 1.5 million women in the UK experience such severe symptoms that their quality of life and interpersonal relationships are greatly affected. Over 35% of these women will seek medical treatment.

Somatic symptoms of premenstrual syndrome include bloating, weight gain, mastalgia, abdominal discomfort and pain, lack of energy, headache and exacerbations of chronic illnesses such as asthma, allergies, epilepsy or migraine. Commonly reported affective changes are dysphoria, irritability, anxiety, tension, aggression, feelings of being unable to cope and a sense of loss of control.

Numerous hypotheses have been advanced to explain PMS, but to date the pathogenesis remains unclear and speculative. Experimental data from randomized controlled trials is sparse when compared to the number of interventions postulated.

Specific to case

PMS is common. However, suicidal ideation/attempts are much less common. It is important that the candidate confirms that this really is PMS by taking a careful history (cyclical pattern) and looking for symptoms more suggestive of a mental illness (depression).

You should communicate in a non-confrontational, empathetic manner but as a clinician with clinical detachment and without appearing to 'indulge' the patient. Reassurance and explanation are an important first step, as well as listening to the patient. Encourage her to try and develop strategies to combat her symptoms when severe (CBT) and accept support from friends/family, and offer simple, proven therapies as first line (vitamin supplements, etc).

In this instance, it is likely that a trial of GnRH-a for 3 months with review will help confirm the diagnosis (distinguish it from mental illness if symptoms resolve) and for longer term treatment consideration should be given to addback HRT (GnRH-a is more efficacious for physical than behavioural symptoms, although the difference is not statistically significant). In reality, if treatment with GnRH-a + addback HRT is successful, then long-term treatment in a 38-year-old woman without future fertility plans would be a hysterectomy + BSO + ERT. In this case an LAVH + BSO may be the best option.

Further reading

Wyatt K. 2003: Premenstrual syndrome. *Clin Evid* **9**:2125–2144.

Station 8 – Vesico-vaginal fistula (Viva, communication, management)

Candidate's instructions

You are the Specialist Registrar on-call for O&G at St Elsewhere Hospital. You have been called to the A&E Department at 8 pm to see a 42-year-old woman who you performed a routine abdominal hysterectomy on 2 weeks ago who has come to Casualty. She is complaining of loss of urinary control and a constant feeling of vaginal wetness necessitating the wearing of sanitary protection.

This is a structured viva. The examiner will ask you a series of questions regarding the management of this woman.

Marks will be awarded for:

Your ability to answer the questions regarding the diagnosis, investigation, treatment and counselling of this patient.

Examiner's instructions

This is a structured viva. You should ask the candidate the questions on your mark sheet. You can prompt the candidate if necessary, but this requirement should be reflected in the global marks awarded.

Questions to be asked:

1. What diagnoses do you suspect?
2. What would your next steps be to confirm or refute the diagnosis?
3. A small vesico-vaginal fistula (VVF) is confirmed on micturating cystogram. The IVU is normal. What would your next steps be in the management of this patient?
4. Now the VVF diagnosis is confirmed, you go to speak to the patient. What would you tell the patient?
5. What would you do after care is taken over by the urologists?

Structured mark sheet

1. What diagnoses do you suspect? [3]

- Urinary tract – vaginal fistula (vesico-vaginal, uretero-vaginal).
- Urinary tract infection.
- Pelvic haematoma/abscess (serous discharge).

0   1   2   3

2. What would your next steps be to confirm or refute the diagnosis? [4]

- Pelvic examination.
- MSU.
- HVS.
- Methylene blue instillation to bladder, visualization ± swab in vagina.
- Admit the patient for further (radiological) investigation unavailable at night.
- Pelvic ultrasound scan.
- Micturating cystogram.
- IVU.

0   1   2   3   4

3. A small vesico-vaginal fistula (VVF) is confirmed on micturating cystogram. The IVU is normal. What would your next steps be in the management of this patient? [2]

- Inform consultant.
- Contact urologists (or urogynaecologist with suitable experience).
- Speak to patient.

0   1   2

4. Now the VVF diagnosis is confirmed, you go to speak to the patient. What would you tell the patient? [6]

- Apologize.
- Infrequent but recognized complication.
- Explain why it occurred – bladder close to vagina anatomically, a misplaced suture may have incorporated the bladder into the vagina, avascular necrosis as a result of infection/haematoma.
- Further management depends upon view of 'bladder specialists' (urologists). They are likely to suggest one of the following:
  - Conservative (cystoscopy/long-term catheter foley/suprapubic urinary catheter);

- Surgery – vaginal; abdominal.
- Either surgical option will require 5–10 days in hospital, long-term catheter (3 months).
- Anticipate good outcome – normal bladder function/continence, although urinary urge symptoms may occur/exacerbate.
- Allow patient to express concerns, uncertainties, do not hide information, be honest, establish a good doctor–patient relationship.

0   1   2   3   4   5   6

5. What would you do after care is taken over by the urologists?   [1]

Follow-up the patient – review regularly as an inpatient, see in gynaecology outpatients ('don't hide').

0   1

Global score   [4]

0   1   2   3   4

Total: **/20**

Case notes

This question not only assesses your clinical experience/knowledge, but also (and more importantly) your communication skills.

With any serious complication, you should inform your consultant immediately. Experience is particularly important in these situations. Older, more experienced consultants will often be approached by their more junior consultant colleagues in infrequent or unusual situations for advice, i.e. 'expert' opinion where 'evidence' is lacking, so you should use the hierarchy also.

Most surgeons will take complications directly related to surgery personally. Despite this you should not 'hide', but keep a high profile and make yourself readily available to the patient and her family. You must give an honest appraisal of the complication (reasons, prognosis) and apologize/empathize.

Try not to contradict what other specialities (in this case urology) may say, but it is reasonable to outline the likely options (if you know them; if not, do not guess!).

Further reading

Hadley HR. 2002: Vesicovaginal fistula. *Curr Urol Rep* **3**:401–407.

Station 9 – Termination of pregnancy, pelvic inflammatory disease and family planning (Counselling, management, viva)

Candidate's instructions

You are about to see Mary Emms, a 25-year-old nulliparous psychology student in your gynaecology outpatient clinic who is requesting a termination of an unwanted pregnancy. She has been on the combined contraceptive pill for the last year and has no medical problems, but feels she cannot cope with an unplanned pregnancy. Her LMP was 11 weeks ago. You examine her and find a 10–12-week sized gravid uterus.

Your task is to conduct an appropriate consultation and explain the management options available. The examiner will then ask a series of questions related to this case.

Marks will be awarded for:

- Appropriate approach to consultation;
- Explaining the management options;
- Your ability to answer the examiner's questions.

Role player's instructions

You are Mary Emms, a 25-year-old nulliparous psychology student. You are very distressed to find yourself pregnant. You are in a steady relationship with your boyfriend and have been taking the COC for the last year, although you forget to take one occasionally. You are adamant you do not want to be pregnant, but are concerned about the physical (particularly the effect on your future fertility) and psychological effects of a TOP. You have discussed things with your boyfriend and you both want to terminate the pregnancy.

Examiner's instructions

Listen to the consultation and award marks according to your mark sheet for how well this is conducted and for the clarity of discussion of appropriate management options. You should then ask the candidate the questions on your mark sheet.

Questions to be asked:

1. She chooses to have a surgical TOP. What investigations do you consider necessary preoperatively and what interventions would you use to reduce TOP-related morbidity?
2. What contraceptive options do you consider appropriate?
3. She chooses to have an IUCD fitted. Three years later her GP sends her to see you as a routine cervical smear reports the presence of actinomyces-like organisms. How do you explain these findings to the patient and what management do you advise?

Structured mark sheet

Consultation and management [6]

- Sensitive, discrete, non-judgemental approach.
- Accurate, impartial verbal information supported by written advice.
- Convey an emphasis on the duty of confidentiality/discretion of healthcare professionals.
- Explore sensitively reasons for 'social' TOP. Ask if they have been discussed with close friends/family.
- Confirm mental capacity, no coercion, not 'knee-jerk' reaction, considered psychological and physical side effects of TOP vs continuing pregnancy (identify risk factors for women likely to experience post-abortion distress – ambivalence before the abortion, lack of a supportive partner, a psychiatric history or membership of a cultural group that considers abortion to be wrong).
- Discuss risks and sequelae of abortion in order to give valid consent:
  - Haemorrhage in 1 in 1000 abortions at this gestation; uterine perforation 1–4 in 1000; cervical trauma 1 in 100; failed abortion and continuing pregnancy (for surgical TOP 2 in 1000; for medical TOP 1–14 in 1000); post-abortion infection: genital tract infection, including pelvic inflammatory disease;
  - Disease of varying degrees of severity, occurs in up to 10% of cases without prophylaxis/bacteriological screening; may be associated with a small increase in the risk of subsequent miscarriage or preterm delivery but reassure no other adverse reproductive outcomes (e.g. infertility); possibly increased psychological sequelae (psychiatric illness or self-harm, although contentious).
- Discuss post-TOP contraception.

- Discuss management options:
  - Surgical TOP – suction (GA or conscious sedation);
  - Medical TOP – mifepristone 200 mg orally, followed 36–48 hours later by misoprostol 800 µg PV, followed by misoprostol 400 µg at 3-hourly intervals, vaginally or orally to a maximum of four further doses.

0   1   2   3   4   5   6

1. She chooses to have a surgical TOP. What investigations do you consider necessary preoperatively and what interventions would you use to reduce TOP-related morbidity? [4]

- Investigations:
  - FBC (Hb);
  - G&S (ABO and Rhesus blood groups, screening for red cell antibodies);
  - Testing for other conditions, e.g. haemoglobinopathies, HIV, and hepatitis B, C (if indicated in the light of clinical features, individual risk factors or local prevalence);
  - Opportunistic cervical screening (if indicated according to cervical cytology screening guidance);
  - USS (confirm gestation, exclude ectopic pregnancy);
  - Lower genital tract swabs [HVS, EC (chlamydia)].
- Interventions:
  - Treat patients with positive lower genital tract swabs; or
  - Universal antibiotics if no screening (metronidazole 1 g PR + doxycycline 100 mg PO bd × 7 days or metronidazole 1 g PR + azithromycin 1 g PO STAT);
  - Cervical preparation (gestation > 10 weeks) – misoprostol 400 mg PV or gemeprost 1 mg 3 hours preoperatively or mifepristone 600 mg PO 36–48 hours preoperatively;
  - Anti-D 250 IU < 72 hours.

0   1   2   3   4

3. What contraceptive options do you consider appropriate? [2]

- IUCD at surgical TOP (?Mirena reduce infection).
- DMPA/implants.
- (Oral daily contraceptives – COC/POP – failed, so probably not best option).

0   1   2

4. She chooses to have an IUCD fitted. Three years later her GP sends her to see you as a routine cervical smear reports the presence of actinomyces-like organisms (ALOs). How do you explain these findings to the patient and what management do you advise? **[4]**

- The presence of ALOs on a cervical smear in a woman with a current IUD requires an assessment to exclude pelvic infection.
- No symptoms/sign of pelvic infection. The Family Planning Association (FPA) recommends that routine removal is not indicated and the woman is counselled regarding the options of removing the IUD, changing the IUD or leaving it in place. It is important to discuss the lack of evidence of harm but that a small increased risk of developing pelvic actinomyces cannot be excluded:
  - If the IUD is removed, a new one can be inserted on the same occasion, ensuring ongoing contraception. The removed IUD does not need to be sent for culture. A cervical smear should be repeated in 3–6 months to check for the presence of persisting ALOs;
  - If the IUD is left in place, adequate follow-up is necessary (e.g. every 6 months). The woman should be warned about symptoms suggesting PID and advised to seek immediate medical advice if these occur. Cervical smears are likely to continue to show the presence of ALOs, and therefore should only be repeated at intervals recommended by the national cervical screening programme.
- Symptoms/signs suggestive of pelvic infection. The FPA recommends that the IUD be removed, the threads sent for culture and the woman treated with an appropriate antibiotic while the results of culture are awaited (a penicillin, tetracycline or erythromycin for at least 2 weeks).

0   1   2   3   4

Global score **[4]**

0   1   2   3   4

Total: **/20**

Case notes

At least one-third of British women will have had an abortion by the time they reach the age of 45 years. Over 98% of induced abortions in Britain are undertaken because of risk to the mental or physical health of the woman or her children.

In these sorts of counselling/management situations where there is a 'finality' of the decision (TOP, sterilization, etc), it is important to allow patients time to reflect on the information discussed at the consultation. The verbal information should be supported by accurate, impartial printed information.

Regarding the abortion decision, clinicians caring for women requesting abortion should try to identify those who require more support in decision-making than can be provided in the routine clinic setting (such as those with a psychiatric history, poor social support or evidence of coercion). Care pathways for additional support, including access to social services, should be available.

If you have a moral objection to TOP, then professional behaviour dictates that you offer referral to another colleague. You should still take an appropriate history to identify medical/surgical risk factors and discuss the potential side effects associated with TOP. You should not give a moral or judgemental opinion in your capacity as a clinician. There are other appropriate forums for this.

Be aware of PID, the evidence-based management thereof and the high prevalence of chlamydial infection in 16–29-year-olds (especially 16–24-year-olds – hence the current national chlamydial opportunistic screening programme). Chlamydia is a serious problem. Around 9% of sexually active young women are likely to be infected and around 70% of infections are asymptomatic, so people do not know that they are infected. The consequences of untreated infection can be serious, and include pelvic inflammatory disease and subsequent infertility. For this reason, those women undergoing TOPs should be screened and/or treated for PID-related organisms.

Do not forget post-TOP contraception to avoid a recurrence. With TOP questions in the OSCE, think contraception and PID in addition to what you would do in a routine consultation.

Further reading

NICE. Clinical Guideline 30 Long-acting reversible contraception 2005 (available at: www.nice.org.uk/page.aspx?o=cg030niceguideline).

Royal College of Obstetricians and Gynaecologists. Setting standards to improve women's health. The Care of Women Requesting Induced Abortion. Evidence-based Clinical Guideline Number 7 (available at: www.rcog.org.uk/resources/Public/pdf/induced_abortionfull.pdf).

Station 10 – Breech presentation (Practical competencies – emergencies)

Candidate's instructions

You have been called to see a 28-year-old woman, who has had two normal vaginal deliveries in the past and now has presented on delivery suite contracting regularly. The midwife attending has found her to be 9 cm dilated with what she thinks is a breech presentation.

The examiner will ask you a series of questions germane to this case.

Marks will be awarded for:

- Managing this situation appropriately;
- Ability to conduct a breech delivery;
- Ability to deal with complications that may arise.

Examiner's instructions

At this station, the candidate will have 14 minutes to discuss and demonstrate the obstetric management of an undiagnosed breech. You should ask the candidate the questions in the order they appear on your mark sheet. You should provide the candidate with the pelvic/fetal model as appropriate. You can prompt the candidate if necessary, but this requirement should be reflected in the marks awarded.

You should have the following equipment:

- Pelvic model;
- 'Fetal' doll.

Questions to be asked:

1. Take me through what you would do?
2. The patient states that she has had two normal deliveries (albeit not breech) before without problems and, as she is almost fully dilated, she would still rather attempt a vaginal delivery. How would you respond to this?
3. She opts for a trial of vaginal delivery. What do you do now?

Give the candidate the fetal doll and you hold the pelvis.

4. The breech has reached the pelvic floor with maternal efforts. Show me how you would conduct the delivery of an extended breech using the doll provided?
5. What would you do in the extreme situation where the head fails to descend into the pelvis once the shoulders have been delivered?

Structured mark sheet

1. Take me through what you would do? [4]

- Attend patient, commence/interpret CTG.
- Determine gestation.
- Speak to patient/review notes.
- Any obstetric risk factors?
- Any relevant maternal medical problems?
- Any management plan? Or is it an undiagnosed breech?
- When last ate/drank?
- Examine the patient (abdominal/vaginal) – confirm breech, position, station, dilatation, exclude footling, size, clinically 'adequate' pelvis.
- [Consider performing USS if skilled – type of breech (extended vs flexed).]
- If footling – C/S.
- If frank (extended)/flexed (complete) breech, then discuss options (trial of vaginal breech vs C/S).

Prompt – role play with me how you would discuss this in your routine practice.

- The best evidence we have from a large study demonstrated that delivery by C/S is safer for the baby (equivalent for the mother).
- Vaginal delivery is three times more likely to result in serious problems to the baby (death, permanent problems, i.e. perinatal mortality, neonatal mortality or serious neonatal morbidity).
- Reassure that the absolute risk of such a problem to the baby is lowish (5%), but again re-emphasize that it is lower (1–2%) with a C/S.
- Risks to mother are low and the same for vaginal delivery and C/S. C/S is associated with longer stay in hospital/recovery time (surgical morbidity).

0   1   2   3   4

2. The patient states that she has had two normal deliveries (albeit not breech) before without problems and, as she is almost fully dilated, she would still rather attempt a vaginal delivery. How would you respond to this? [1]

- Agree – that this is fine and her choice but …
- Explain that although you would intuitively expect, given her past obstetric history and advanced stage of labour, that successful, safe breech delivery would be more likely than not, the main risk/most hazardous part of a breech delivery relates to the aftercoming head (i.e. head getting stuck). Thus, C/S must still be considered safer for the baby.

0   1

3. She opts for a trial of vaginal delivery. What do you do now? [2]

- Call consultant/summon more experienced help.
- Continuous EFM (CTG).
- Gain IV access.
- Inform anaesthetist on-call – will need to be available at delivery.
- Discuss analgesia – recommend epidural (although not essential and there may not be time) to allow for obstetric manipulations that may be required.
- Delivery in theatre preferable (especially if no regional anaesthesia), but adequately equipped delivery room with rapid access to theatre acceptable.

0   1   2

Give the candidate the fetal doll and you hold the pelvis.

4. The breech has reached the pelvic floor with maternal efforts. Show me how you would conduct the delivery of an extended breech using the doll provided? [8]

- General principle = 'hands off', i.e. don't interfere. Allow most, if not all, the delivery to occur spontaneously (often achievable in multiparous women).
- Supine (lithotomy) vs upright position (use the one you are most familiar with).
- Empty bladder.
- Consider episiotomy (may not be necessary as multiparous) when anus visible over the vaginal fourchette (protect the fetal bottom with your left hand).
- Observe ± guide (do not pull) the breech upward as it 'crowns'. If the sacrum does not rotate from the sacral lateral position to an anterior position, then help rotate it (thumbs on fetal spine, fingers on iliac crests).

- Deliver the extended legs by flexion of the knee joints (finger in popliteal fossa) and extension/abduction of the hip joints and 'walk the legs out'.
- Bring a loop of cord down (take it off tension, avoid tearing).
- Support the breech baby and wrap in a towel to keep warm (allow the baby to 'hang' down so gravity aids delivery).
- As the anterior shoulder scapula tip ('wing') becomes visible with maternal pushing, deliver one arm by running a finger over the shoulder and down to the elbow to deliver the arm (sweep across the chest). Repeat on the other side (may need gently to rotate the baby to aid access).
- If arms extended over the fetal head, then perform Lovsett's manoeuvre (thumbs on sacrum, rotate fetal back through 180° until the posterior arm lies anteriorly. The exposed elbow is now below the symphysis pubis and that arm and hand can be delivered by sweeping it across the fetal chest. Repeat in reverse to deliver the other arm. (Complication: 'nuchal arm' – flexed at elbow, extended at shoulder and behind the fetal head – modified Lovsett's).
- Support the baby (allow the baby to 'hang' down so gravity aids delivery) until nape of neck visible (descent of the head into the pelvis).
- Paediatrician present to suction mouth and pharynx on the perineum prior to complete delivery of the head.
- Deliver the head (have an assistant scrubbed ready to help, understand importance of flexing the fetal head):
  - Mauriceau–Smellie–Veit manoeuvre. 'Traction in axis of birth canal + flexion' – support fetus on right forearm (horizontal, above horizontal); middle finger gently in fetal mouth and ring/index fingers on malar eminences or fetal shoulders; traction is then applied to flex and deliver whilst simultaneously using the left hand to exert pressure upward and posteriorly on the fetal occiput to encourage flexion ± suprapubic pressure (further flexion and descent);
  - Burns Marshall. Grasp the fetal ankles (usually assistant) and raise vertically above the mother's abdomen – promotes flexion of the head – spontaneous delivery or middle finger gently in fetal mouth and ring/index fingers on malar eminences to aid further flexion in the AP diameter;
  - Forceps. Grasp the fetal ankles (usually assistant) and raise vertically above the mother's abdomen, apply mid-cavity forceps (i.e. long shank) below the fetal body – promotes flexion of the head – spontaneous delivery or middle finger gently in fetal mouth and ring/index fingers on malar eminences to aid further flexion in the AP diameter.

0   1   2   3   4   5   6   7   8

5. What would you do in the extreme situation where the head fails to descend into the pelvis once the shoulders have been delivered? [1]

- Turn fetal body sideways and apply suprapubic pressure to flex and descend the head in conjunction with the operator's finger in the fetal mouth.
- Weighted speculum in vagina (allow baby to breathe) and symphysiotomy.
- Push fetal body upwards and perform C/S.

0   1

Global score [4]

0   1   2   3   4

Total: /20

Case notes

The incidence of breech presentation is about 20% at 28 weeks. Most of the fetuses turn spontaneously, so the incidence at term is 3–4%. It has been widely recognized that there is higher perinatal mortality and morbidity with breech presentation, due principally to prematurity, congenital malformations and birth asphyxia or trauma.

The Term Breech Trial (an international multicentre RCT of planned vaginal delivery versus planned elective caesarean section for the uncomplicated term breech) recommended that 'the best method of delivering a term frank or complete breech singleton is by planned LSCS'. Its key findings were:

- The overall risk of perinatal death for the term frank/complete breech fetus with planned caesarean birth was reduced by 75% (RR 0.23; CI 0.07–0.8);
- Perinatal mortality, neonatal mortality or serious neonatal morbidity was significantly lower for the planned caesarean section group than for the planned vaginal birth group [17 of 1039 (1.6%) vs 52 of 1039 (5.0%); relative risk 0.33 (95% CI 0.19–0.56); P < 0.0001].
- There were no differences between groups in terms of maternal mortality or serious maternal morbidity [41 of 1041 (3.9%) vs 33 of 1042 (3.2%); 1.24 (0.79–1.95); P = 0.35].

At this station you need to convey your clinical maturity in dealing with this unplanned situation. This requires a fundamental awareness of the risks breech presentation in labour presents, a basic understanding of evidence supporting current practice and good communication skills to allow balanced counselling and the acquisition of informed consent.

If you have practised mainly in the UK, then your experience of assisted vaginal breech delivery is likely to be small. However, situations such as the one presented in this case may arise and, as the RCOG guidance (see Further reading) suggests, it remains important that clinicians and hospitals are prepared for vaginal breech delivery. You should not come across as 'cavalier', but show a prudent, cautious approach. This means always informing your senior (hopefully more experienced!) colleagues, including the consultant on-call, of potentially complicated deliveries, even if you feel confident in their management. Such deliveries include breech presentation and twin deliveries.

An excellent candidate will not only be aware of the techniques described for delivery of the aftercoming head, but also the manoeuvres required when complications arise (extended arms, nuchal arm, head entrapment).

Further reading

Hannah ME, Hannah WJ, Hewson SA, 2000: Planned caesarean section versus planned vaginal birth for breech presentation at term: a randomized multicentre trial. Term Breech Trial Collaborative Group. *Lancet* **356**:1375–1383.

Johanson RB. 2003: Breech and external cephalic version: In: Johanson R, Cox C, Grady K, Howell C, eds. *Managing Obstetric Emergencies and Trauma*. The MOET Course Manual. London: RCOG Press, Chapter 23.

RCOG Green Top Guideline. The Management of Breech Presentation (20) – Apr 2001 (available at: www.rcog.org.uk/index.asp?PageID=513).

Station 11 – Unstable lie and cord prolapse (Viva, management, practical competencies)

Candidate's instructions

At this station you will have 14 minutes to answer questions about the obstetric management of an unstable lie.

This is a structured viva. The examiner will ask you a series of questions about issues relating to the management of an unstable lie in pregnancy.

Marks will be awarded for:

- Your ability to answer questions about the obstetric management of an unstable lie;
- Your ability to deal with complications related to an unstable lie.

Examiner's instructions

At this station, the candidate will have 14 minutes to discuss the obstetric management of an unstable lie. You should ask the candidate the questions in the order they appear on your mark sheet.

Questions to be asked:

1. What is an unstable lie and what factors may predispose to or cause an unstable lie?
2. How would you manage a woman who is para 3, all normal vaginal deliveries, with an unstable lie discovered in your antenatal clinic at 38 weeks' gestation, and justify your management?
3. She refuses hospital admission because of childcare commitments. What would you do now?
4. She arrives on labour ward 1 week later with uterine contractions. The SHO examining her has diagnosed a transverse lie clinically and a portable scan has confirmed this, with the head in the right flank and the back is posterior. Whilst waiting to be seen in the triage area of admissions, she ruptures her membranes. The emergency buzzer goes as the midwife looking after her has seen the cord dangling down from the vagina. You attend immediately. What do you do now?
5. Describe how you would perform the caesarean section.
6. What would you do if you inadvertently deliver an arm instead of a foot during attempted breech extraction?

Structured mark sheet

1. What is an unstable lie and what factors may predispose to or cause an unstable lie? [3]

- Definition:
  - When the presentation of the fetus changes day to day, the lie is said to be unstable;
  - The fetal lie describes the relationship of the fetus to the long axis of the mother;
  - Synonymous with *oblique* (an anatomical relationship in which the fetal axis crosses the maternal axis at an angle other than a right angle) or *transverse* lie (an anatomical relationship in which the long axis of the fetus lies at right angles to the long axis of the mother).
- Causes:
  - Grand multiparity (flaccid uterus/lax and pendulous abdominal wall);
  - Contracted pelvis;
  - Polyhydramnios;
  - Prematurity;
  - Subseptate uterus;
  - Placenta praevia;
  - Pelvic tumours such as fibroids and ovarian cysts.

0   1   2   3

2. How would you manage a woman who is para 3, all normal vaginal deliveries, with an unstable lie discovered in your antenatal clinic at 38 weeks' gestation and justify your management? [4]

- Ultrasound scan (placental position, uterine anomalies, pelvic tumours, fetal anomalies, define presentation, cord presentation).
- Admit (risk of cord prolapse if SROM).
- Explain diagnosis and rationale for hospital admission given the serious potential sequelae to the baby.
- Management according to cause. In general, if not placenta praevia, cord presentation or anatomical obstruction to fetal head engagement (these require C/S), then:
  - Vaginal examination (Bishop's score – help decide if IOL feasible);
  - Expectant (daily examination, await reversion of lie to longitudinal for 48 hours, then allow home for IOL at 41 weeks);
  - IOL [stabilizing induction (at 41 weeks preferable)] – IV access, ECV and controlled ARM in theatre on labour ward and commence oxytoxin

infusion, anaesthetist – avoids surgical morbidity associated with C/S; if cervix is favourable, then early IOL does not waste time; may reduce risk of uterine rupture compared to expectant;
- Caesarean section at 39 weeks (remove risks of cord prolapse during labour and uterine rupture).

0   1   2   3   4

3. She refuses hospital admission because of childcare commitments. What would you do now? [2]

- Document that you have explained the risks and that the mother has the mental capacity to make an informed choice.
- Reinforce that if she changes her mind or can make arrangements for childcare, then she can return for recommended hospital admission at any time.
- Advise her to return immediately if she experiences uterine contractions, vaginal bleeding or fluid leakage (suspected SROM).

0   1   2

4. She arrives on labour ward 1 week later with uterine contractions. The SHO examining her has diagnosed a transverse lie clinically and a portable scan has confirmed this, with the head in the right flank and the back is posterior. Whilst waiting to be seen in the triage area of admissions, she ruptures her membranes. The emergency buzzer goes as the midwife looking after her has seen the cord dangling down from the vagina. You attend immediately. What do you do now? [4]

- Vaginal examination.
- Assess cervical dilatation and cord pulsation.
- Put patient in knee–chest or Trendelenburg position.
- Replace umbilical cord back into the vagina (prevent asphyxia from spasm of the cord vessels when exposed to cold or manipulation).
- Manually elevate the presenting part above the pelvic inlet (prevent asphyxia from mechanical cord compression between the presenting part and bony pelvis) or insert Foley urinary catheter and fill the bladder with 500 ml of physiological saline and clamp (release at skin incision at C/S).
- Simultaneously ask the midwife to obtain a Doppler FHR ± USS.
- If fully dilated and vertex presentation, consider instrumental vaginal delivery (ventouse if unengaged head).
- Transfer to theatre for an emergency caesarean section.

0   1   2   3   4

5. Describe how you would perform the caesarean section [2]

- General anaesthesia preferable for speed (unless maternal risk factors). Consider regional block if bladder filled and CTG normal.
- LSCS generally possible at term with recent SROM.
- Consider classical approach if minimal liquor left as back down, transverse lie can be difficult.
- Deliver baby through uterine incision by ECV or internal podalic rotation and gentle breech extraction.

0   1   2

6. What would you do if you inadvertently deliver an arm instead of a foot during attempted breech extraction? [1]
Replace the hand/arm and try again to locate the foot/feet.

0   1

Global score [4]

0   1   2   3   4

Total: **/20**

Case notes

There are no definitive guidelines about the management of an unstable lie. In practice these tend to occur in multiparous women and, in the absence of any obstruction to engagement of the fetal head, the lie normally corrects with the onset of labour contractions and as normal labour progresses. However, given the potential for fetal demise as a result of cord prolapse, the stakes are high and so caution is prudent. Generally, in a woman without a history of preterm delivery, these women can be managed as outpatients until 36–38 weeks with the proviso that they should be admitted if there are any signs of labour.

Suspect an unstable (oblique/transverse) lie in women with risk factors and on examination if the shape of the abdomen on inspection appears wider laterally (if transverse), the SFH may be reduced, using standard Leopold's manoeuvres the fetal pole will be detected laterally or obliquely, not overlying the pelvic brim. Digital cervical exam will confirm no presenting part – usually shoulder (lying over pelvic brim). However, it is best to defer vaginal examination until a USS confirms your abdominal findings and excludes placenta praevia.

In clinical practice, patients do not always want to take our advice. As long as the woman has the competence (i.e. capacity) to withhold consent (i.e. she has understood what has been said), then she is within her rights to do so (i.e. she needs capacity but not good judgement!). However, a mature clinician will not be offended by this 'slight', but will respect her views, document things carefully and offer review and access to services. It is important, however, that the patient is left in no doubt about what you consider to be the best management in her case and what the potential complications are, which will be her responsibility. You can still maintain a good rapport without 'agreeing' with the patient or being manipulated around to her way of thinking. Role players at OSCE counselling stations may be primed to do this!

Cord prolapse complicates 0.2% of all births, but the incidence will be higher in an unstable lie. This is an emergency situation where speed is essential as stillbirth and neonatal morbidity is significantly related to the time interval between diagnosis and delivery. You should be familiar with the emergency drill.

Further reading

Goswami K. 2003: Prolapsed umbilical cord. In: Johanson R, Cox C, Grady K, Howell C, eds. *Managing Obstetric Emergencies and Trauma*. The MOET Course Manual. London: RCOG Press, Chapter 18.

Station 12 – Miscarriage (Counselling, management, data interpretation)

Candidate's instructions

You are about to see Mrs Jane Paige, a 26-year-old nulliparous flight attendant who presented with an 8-week history of amenorrhoea, a positive urinary pregnancy test and light blood-stained vaginal discharge. This is her third first-trimester miscarriage in the last 2 years. She has no past medical history of note.

Examination revealed a slim woman, with normal vital signs, no abdominal tenderness. On pelvic examination a closed external cervical os was seen with no intravaginal blood visible. She has just returned from the ultrasound department with the following report:

Early pregnancy scan: Transabdominal/transvaginal pelvic ultrasound
Jane Paige   **DOB 19-09-1979**
Source: Early Pregnancy Assessment Unit
Indication: Threatened miscarriage ? viability

Gestation sac:	Seen	Endometrium:	Thickened
Position:	Normal	Bleed:	No
Size:	Not performed	Masses:	No
Volume:	10 ml	Free fluid:	No
Yolk sac:	Seen	Right ovary:	Not performed
Fetus:	Seen	Left ovary:	Not performed
Heart:	Not seen		
CRL:	9 mm		

Your task is to explain the diagnosis to the patient and to address any concerns the patient may have. You then need to discuss appropriate management options.

Marks will be awarded for:

- Explaining the diagnosis;
- Adequately and sensitively addressing the patient's concerns;
- Discussing appropriate management options.

Role player's instructions

You are Jane Paige, a married 26-year-old air hostess. You discovered you were pregnant when you were late for your period and did a pregnancy test 3 weeks ago. You think you are about 8 weeks' pregnant.

You noticed some light bleeding 2 days ago, which stained your underwear. You had no pain, but you became extremely anxious as you are desperate for a baby. You have had two early miscarriages (at 6 and 10 weeks of pregnancy) in the last 2 years. One of these pregnancies miscarried naturally and the other required an operation called a 'D&C'.

You have just returned from the scan department very upset because the lady who performed the scan abruptly told you that 'she could see the fetus, but no heart beat was seen'.

Questions you need to ask during the consultation:

- What did the scan lady mean when she said that she could not see the baby's heart beat?
- Why has it happened this time?
- Why has it happened for a third time?
- Is it my fault?
- What treatment would you advise me to have doctor?

Structured mark sheet

Explain diagnosis and address patient's concerns [8]

- Early intrauterine pregnancy with a non-viable fetus:
  - Use the term 'silent miscarriage' (recommended alternatives 'delayed miscarriage'/'early fetal demise'; missed abortion no longer recommended);
  - Use simple language, e.g. a miscarriage is the early loss of a pregnancy.
- Put in context. *'Unfortunately miscarriage is common and occurs in around 1 in 4 pregnancies. Miscarriages can occur at various times in early pregnancy, but most commonly within the first 12 weeks. Your baby appears to have stopped developing after 7 weeks.'*
- Identify and address patient's concerns:
  - Why miscarriage? It cannot be said for certainty why a miscarriage occurs, but the most common reason is that the embryo (fertilized egg) does not develop normally;
  - Is it my fault? Reassure the patient that, *'Your miscarriage is unlikely to have happened because of anything you did or didn't do. Sadly, it's just very common'*;
  - Why a third miscarriage? *'Early miscarriage is sadly common and the chances are you will successfully carry a future pregnancy to term. Around 1 in 100 women will lose three or more early pregnancies and we call this 'recurrent miscarriage'. This is about three times more than you would expect to happen just by chance, so it seems that for some women there must be a specific reason for their losses. For others, however, no underlying problem can be identified; their repeated miscarriages may be due to chance alone'*;
  - Why does recurrent miscarriage occur? *'Despite careful investigations, we often cannot find a reason to explain recurrent miscarriage. A number of things may play a part in recurrent miscarriage. It is a complicated problem and more research is still needed.'* Potential causes include (use simple lay language to explain): genetic factors/abnormalities in the

embryo; immunological – autoimmune factors; anatomical – uterine abnormalities; hormonal (endocrine) – PCO, hyperprolactinaemia, diabetes, thyroid problems; infections; blood conditions (thrombophilias).

- Empathy/attend to patient:
  - Acknowledge her grief – *'I'm very sorry. …; It must be a distressing time for you and your partner. …; Its OK to be upset/angry. …; Do you need time alone. …; Do you want anyone else here?'*
  - Offer further support – written information, support group numbers (e.g. The Miscarriage Association).

0   1   2   3   4   5   6   7   8

Discuss management options [8]

- Ascertain what happened with her two previous miscarriages. This gives a starting point of knowledge and her perceptions about previous experiences which are likely to affect her choices.
- Expectant (conservative):
  - Explain what it involves – allow home, await events naturally to occur;
  - Explain what to expect in terms of symptoms (bleeding/pain);
  - Reassure, send home with analgesics, contact for advice, can change mind;
  - Follow-up with USS to check resolution;
  - Advantages – 'natural', safe, no intervention;
  - Disadvantages – may take up to 6 weeks (distressing/inconvenient); may get infection; may fail – require medical ERPC/surgical ERPC.
- Medical:
  - Explain what it involves – allow home vs inpatient admission (depends on regimen), await events to then occur naturally;
  - Explain what to expect in terms of symptoms (bleeding/pain);
  - Reassure, analgesics, contact for advice, can change mind;
  - Follow-up with USS to check resolution;
  - Advantages – safe, avoids need for surgical intervention, anaesthetic/ surgical complications;
  - Disadvantages – may need repeating, may take up to 6 weeks (distressing/inconvenient), may get infection, side effects (GIT), may fail to complete the ERPC – require repeat medical ERPC or recourse to surgical ERPC.
- Surgical:
  - Explain what it involves – admission, type of anaesthesia, potential risks (bleeding, infection, perforation);

- – Advantages – rapid 'closure', safe, no need for further investigations (USS, etc), minimal further problems with bleeding or pain (after initial post-operative cramps);
  - – Disadvantages – potential surgical/anaesthetic complications, hospital admission required.
- Which one would you advise doctor?
  - – Explain that ultimately it is her decision;
  - – As patient is fit and well and early loss, then surgical/anaesthetic risks are minimal, so many women value a quick resolution allowing them time to grieve/recover;
  - – Medical ERPC is also very effective and generally allows a quick resolution without need for surgery/anaesthetic, so if worried about surgery then medical ERPC represents a good compromise between 'natural' and 'surgical';
  - – Conservative – highly effective in women with 'incomplete miscarriage' (pregnancy partly expelled), but completing miscarriage naturally with a 'silent miscarriage' generally takes longer (3 6 weeks) and effectiveness is reduced. So if unsure, or worried about further bleeding/pain/support at home, then not the best option.

0   1   2   3   4   5   6   7   8

Global score

0   1   2   3   4

Total: **/20**

Case notes

The subject matter in this OSCE station will be familiar to you. However, questions examining common situations paradoxically can be badly answered due to a lack of care and attention on the candidate's part. Think how you would handle the situation on a day-to-day basis. Display your comprehensive knowledge of the management options available, but do not simply regurgitate it as if from a textbook. You are not following a 'recipe' and the good candidate will individualize their approach, use clear, simple language, pick up on verbal and non-verbal prompts and offer guidance.

You need to show that you are aware that patients who are distressed may be vulnerable and require careful counselling, with opportunities for rest, reflection and 'breathing space', and should not be cajoled into a management decision they regret later. In real life, how you handle these sensitive issues in emotionally distressed patients will impact on her and her partner's recovery and avoid complaints.

Common mistakes include:

- Not listening to the patient (spend 90% of the time talking) and failing to pick up on verbal/non-verbal prompts. This results in the candidate 'bombarding' the patient with information.
- Giving facts and figures which either bamboozle the patient or are presented in such a way that the patient cannot interpret them (remember the patient is not a statistic, but an individual – ball park figures are acceptable, but keep referencing these back to the patient's particular circumstances).
- Not allowing patients to express their views/preferences – this is essential where a choice in management approach is available.

Overall between 70% and 90% of women are expected to have a complete miscarriage with medical management. Non-surgical approaches to treating miscarriage are more successful for incomplete miscarriages compared with silent miscarriages. This is especially true with conservative (expectant) treatment.

Most medical miscarriage regimens utilize the oral antiprogesterone tablets (mifepristone) to 'prime' the uterus so it is more responsive to the prostaglandin tablets (vaginal and oral) given in hospital 36–48 hours later. In this way the miscarriage is completed more quickly and more effectively. However, up to one-third of women will bleed or miscarry at home in the priming phase. This should be explained to the patient when discussing medical miscarriage.

Note should be made on early pregnancy scans – a repeat scan must be arranged in 7–10 days time if the sac volume is < 4 ml; CRL < 6 mm with no FH; any doubt exists about viability; a TVS has not been performed.

Further reading

RCOG Green Top Guideline. The Management of Early Pregnancy Loss (25) – Oct 2000 (available at: www.rcog.org.uk/index.asp?PageID=515).

RCOG Green Top Guideline. The Investigation and Treatment of Couples with Recurrent Miscarriage (17) – May 2003 (available at: www.rcog.org.uk/index.asp?PageID=538).

12 Practice circuit 2

- Duration – 3 hours
- Structure – 12 stations × 15 minutes
- Additional information: The bell will sound 1 minute before the conclusion of the station (i.e. at 14 minutes) to allow 1 minute for the examiner to complete the mark sheet and during which time you will move to the next station and begin to read the relevant information.

In addition to questions, detailed structured mark sheets and case notes are provided.

Station 1 – Labour ward prioritization (Preparatory station)

Candidate's instructions

You are the Obstetric SpR on-call for the labour ward. You have arrived for handover at 08:30. There are 10 women currently on the labour ward and a brief summary of each patient is given on the labour ward board.

The staff available to you today are:

- A 3rd year career SHO in O&G;
- A 3rd year SpR in anaesthetics;
- Six midwives JW is in charge, JW and KF can insert IV lines and suture; BS and RJ can suture; AB and CD are newly qualified and cannot suture or site IV lines;
- The consultant has been called to the gynaecology theatre and is dealing with a ruptured ectopic. He is available by phone but is likely to be busy for the next hour.

Read the board carefully. You have 15 minutes to prepare for this station.

Your job is efficiently to manage the labour ward. At the next station you will meet the examiner with whom you will discuss your decisions and your reasoning.

Marks will be awarded for:

Your ability to answer the set questions about the management of the first and second stages of labour, displaying sound judgement, good decision-making and the ability to prioritize cases.

TABLE 12.1

Room	Name	Parity	Gestation	Liquor	Epidural	Syntocinon	Comments	Midwife
1	Robinson	1	40	Intact	No	No	Had prostin pessary at 22:00 last night. IOL for pregnancy-induced hypertension. Previous caesarean section. 2 cm dilated at 06:00, contracting 2 in 10 with a normal CTG. Patient requesting a caesarean section	AB
2	Neville	2	28	Intact	No	No	Dr to see. Arrived on labour ward at 07:30. Contracting 3 in 10, requesting pethidine	CD
3	Cole	1	39	–	No	–	Delivered at 07:00. Retained placenta. Awaiting manual removal in theatre	BS
4 HDU	Terry	2	37	–	–	–	Forceps delivery at 02:00. Had PPH of 2000 ml due to an atonic uterus. Required EUA and Rusch balloon to tamponade bleeding. CVP line and arterial line in situ. Hb 8.3 g/dl at 06:00 after completing 3rd unit of blood. Minimal vaginal blood loss now and observations stable	KF
5 HDU	Ferdinand	1	32	–	–	–	Delivered at 20:00 last night by caesarean section for severe pre-eclampsia. Feeling breathless with O_2 saturations of 91% on 2 L oxygen. Urine output 100 ml since midnight. BP is 160/100	KF
6	Gerrard	0	34	Meconium	No	No	Undiagnosed breech at 8 cm dilated. Just arrived on labour ward from home	BS
7	Beckham	0	39	Meconium	Yes	Yes	Fully dilated since 06:00. Pushing for 1 hour. No vertex visible. CTG variable decelerations with good recovery to normal baseline heart rate	RJ
8	Lampard	0	41	Clear	Yes	Yes	6 cm at 23:00 and 02:00. Syntocinon commenced at 02:30. Vaginal assessment at 05:30 was still 6 cm. Normal CTG	RJ
9	Owen	0	36	Intact	No	No	Twins ceph/breech in ? early labour. Cervix closed at 01:00. Contractions 1 in 15. Normal CTG	AB
10	Rooney	1	42	–	–	–	Normal vaginal delivery at 08:00. Bleeding lightly from a second degree tear. Awaiting suturing	CD

Station 2 – Labour ward prioritization (Prioritization/management)

Your job is efficiently to manage the labour ward and at this station you will discuss your decisions and your reasoning for them with the examiner.

Marks will be awarded for:

Your ability to answer the set questions about the management of the first and second stages of labour, displaying sound judgement, good decision-making and the ability to prioritize cases.

Examiner's instructions

Candidates have 14 minutes to explain the following:

- The tasks that need doing on the delivery suite;
- The order in which they should be done;
- The staff who should be allocated to each.

Tasks to be performed

TABLE 12.2

Room 1	Midwife can reassure patient that she has asked for a medical review regarding her request. Explain that labour ward busy so may be a short time. Optimize analgesia, keep NBM. Ask midwife colleague to site IV access and FBC/G&S
Room 2	Threatened PTL – needs urgent medical review/VE (+ fibronectin) and CTG. Decision can then be made regarding mode of delivery, tocolysis and steroids. Inform paediatricians/NNU re space + ITU
Room 3	Midwife to site IV access, FBC, G&S, check vital signs and observe for bleeding to assess urgency of medical review (VE, oxytocin) and intervention/consent. As will need to go to theatre for manual removal of placenta (MRP) keep NBM, IV fluids and prepare for theatre (antacids, etc)
Room 4	Midwife to record vital signs/observations on HDU chart. Although high risk patient requiring medical review, she is stable now
Room 5	Urgent medical review required of a high risk patient by the whole on-call team as likely renal impairment and pulmonary oedema complicating pre-eclampsia. However, delegate initial review of fluids and investigations to anaesthetic SpR in view of other priorities. Will require systemic examination, FBC, clotting, PET profile, ABG and CXR. Needs O_2 dose increasing, fluid management and antihypertensive review (likely needs fluid restriction + diuretics) and nephrology opinion guided by the results

TABLE 12.2 *(continued)*

Room 6	Urgent medical review (including antenatal history) as active labour and delivery imminent. Needs VE to confirm dilatation/progress and exclude footling breech, and obtain CTG. Need to discuss mode of delivery and consent as appropriate. Ask midwife to keep NBM, site IV access and do FBC/G&S
Room 7	Although nulliparous, she should have delivered by now. In view of possible fetal compromise (meconium + abnormal CTG) she needs urgent review/CTG. PA/VE examinations to ascertain feasibility of instrumental delivery in room/theatre + caesarean section. Urgency depends upon CTG – if Room 2 or 6 need to go first then consider asking SHO to do FBS to exclude fetal acidosis/hypoxia and 'buy time'. If needs CS, stop oxytocin whilst awaiting theatre
Room 8	Ask midwife to do VE to check progress. If failure to progress (secondary arrest), i.e. not 8 cm dilated, then ask her to stop oxytocin, keep NBM, IV access, FBC/G&S and prepare for theatre (antacids, etc). Ask midwife to explain situation to patient and medical review will follow
Room 9	Although high risk pregnancy, it does not sound like this twin pregnancy is in active labour and there is no fetal compromise. Keep on LW and review later. May be able to go to the antenatal ward to await events
Room 10	Midwife to assess degree of bleeding/urgency of vaginal suturing. CD to ask JW to delegate another midwife to suture

Priority of tasks

There may not be total agreement with these suggestions. The candidate needs to demonstrate confidence in making rationale and safe decisions. A degree of flexibility is allowed in the marking.

- Urgent review: Rooms 2, 5, 6 and 7
- Semi-urgent review: Rooms 3, 4 and 8
- Routine review: Rooms 1, 9 and 10

Personnel

All these cases, with the exception of Room 10, will require a medical review involving the candidate as the SpR. However, in view of the other pressing priorities initial delegation of staff should be as follows:

Room 1	Midwife – ask JW or KF to site lines
Room 2	Urgent SHO
Room 3	SHO
Room 4	SpR
Room 5	Urgent anaesthetic SpR followed by O&G SpR
Room 6	Urgent SpR

Room 7   Urgent SpR
Room 8   SHO/SpR
Room 9   Midwife (not AB or CD)
Room 10   Midwife – change CD for BS or RJ

Structured mark sheet

Room 1	0	1	2	3	4
Room 2	0	1	2	3	4
Room 3	0	1	2	3	4
Room 4	0	1	2	3	4
Room 5	0	1	2	3	4
Room 6	0	1	2	3	4
Room 7	0	1	2	3	4
Room 8	0	1	2	3	4
Room 9	0	1	2	3	4
Room 10	0	1	2	3	4

Gross mark: /40 × ½

Total: /20

Case notes

This station is an opportunity to display your day-to-day labour ward management skills. The OSCE is trying to identify those candidates with sound clinical skills and commensurate experience rather than 'bookworms'. Those of you who are or have been in busy clinical jobs should look forward to these stations, as they are an opportunity to 'get away from the books' and demonstrate your abilities. Those of you who have limited clinical experience should not panic. Have confidence as you obviously have the right knowledge to get this far, but practise/role play these types of stations with colleagues when preparing for the OSCE.

Relax to some degree as there is some flexibility in approaching clinical scenarios and your answer does not have to agree exactly with the stylized mark sheet. However, a clear, rational chain of thought should come across and you should convey confidence and a sense of urgency in your decision-making. As the SpR on-call, you should take on the most challenging situations and delegate accordingly. (Note: You are lucky that you have a relatively experienced SHO who you can deploy as a 'junior registrar'!)

It is acceptable to add caveats such as, *'Ideally I would like to review this woman myself, but given the business/more pressing priorities I would delegate so and so ...'* or *'Although my consultant is tied up I would want to inform him of the work load and activity on labour ward and my plans to deal with it'*. Obviously a safe candidate would inform their senior colleagues, but the aim of these stations is to test *your* abilities. It is acceptable to weigh up the options out loud and to mention informing your boss, *but* you need to come across as decisive (and not unsure), confident (but not cavalier or arrogant), calm (but not without a sense of urgency) and able effectively to delegate (but not be lazy or alternatively obsessive).

Where mark schemes offer flexibility, the examiner's assessment of how you come across is important. Remember: *convey calmness, confidence and decisiveness alongside thoughtfulness and safety. Give the impression that you deal with this workload day to day and that you take your job seriously.*

Station 3 – Breaking bad news (Communication, counselling)

Candidate's instructions

You are about so see Amy Samrice, a 48-year-old teacher, in your gynaecology clinic to give her the results of her recent investigations.

She presented to you 2 weeks ago with peri-menopausal bleeding. Clinical examination at the time suggested that the uterus was enlarged and immobile and you could see a mass within the uterus on pelvic ultrasound. You arranged an urgent MRI scan and performed an endometrial biopsy. You arranged to review Mrs Samrice in 2 weeks with the results. Unfortunately the results have confirmed a high grade endometrial adenocarcinoma and the MRI shows invasion of the full myometrial thickness, including the uterine scrosa.

Your task is to break the news and explain the diagnosis.

Marks will be awarded for:

- Breaking bad news appropriately;
- Explaining the diagnosis and implications;
- Responding to the patient's questions and concerns;
- Appropriate conduct of the consultation.

Role player's instructions

You are Amy Samrice, a 48-year-old teacher. You are divorced and have a daughter who is about to go off to university.

You have always had heavy periods but noticed recently that they have become heavier and more erratic. You have felt increasingly tired and do not have much appetite; your daughter commented that you are losing weight. Your GP thought it was all 'due to the change' (i.e. the menopause). He referred you to the hospital for investigation and treatment.

You are expecting to get the results of your tests today and to receive some treatment for your heavy periods. You are not expecting to receive any bad news.

On receiving the news of advanced endometrial cancer (cancer of the lining of the womb):

- Act shocked and devastated – totally unprepared;
- Be uncommunicative initially (silence for a minute of two);
- Denial initially – 'It can't be true'; 'It must be a mistake', 'I can't believe I'm hearing this, I thought it was a routine appointment for menopausal problems', etc;
- Regain composure, although remain tearful/upset and ask the following questions in any order:
  – Am I going to die?
  – How long am I going to live for?
  – What am I going to tell my daughter?
  – What treatment will I need?

Feel free to ask anything else you feel in keeping with the situation.

Examiner's instructions

Candidates have 14 minutes to demonstrate the following:

- Ability to break bad news appropriately;
- Ability to explain the diagnosis and implications;
- Ability to respond to the patient's questions and concerns;
- Appropriate conduct of the consultation.

Structured mark sheet

Communication – Breaking the bad news [4]

- Introduction – greet, introduce, eye contact.

- Set the scene – summarize the situation to date and assess the patient's understanding first: what the patient already knows, is thinking or has been told.
- Break the bad news (share the information):
  - Do not delay in giving the information but give 'warning notes' first that difficult information is coming, e.g. preface with *'I'm afraid that the tests have shown. ...'*, *'I'm afraid it looks more serious than we had hoped ...'* or *'I'm terribly sorry to give you this news but the tests have shown ...'*;
  - Give basic information, simply and honestly;
  - Repeat important points;
  - Do not give too much information too early, thereby overwhelming the patient;
  - Give information in small 'chunks' to aid understanding;
  - Watch the pace of information giving – check repeatedly for understanding and feelings as you proceed;
  - Use language carefully with regard given to the patient's intelligence, reactions, emotions: avoid jargon.

0   1   2   3   4

Explain diagnosis and implications [4]

- Diagnosis – cancer. The tumour has invaded the uterine serosa (the layer of tissue that surrounds the outside of the uterus); Stage III (this stage means the disease is more advanced and that cancer cells have spread to other parts of the pelvis; IIIA – means that it is likely that cancer cells have escaped into the abdomen).
- Prognosis – Stage III may not be curable but 3 in every 10 (30%) patients live for at least 5 years after diagnosis with this stage of womb cancer.

0   1   2   3   4

Responding to patient's questions and concerns [4]

- Management and support: surgery (TAH + BSO + biopsies); radiotherapy; possibly chemotherapy; regular follow-up over number of years.
- Planning and support:
  - Having identified all the patient's specific concerns, offer specific help by breaking down overwhelming feelings into manageable concerns;
  - Identify a plan for what is to happen next;
  - Give a broad time frame for what may lie ahead;
  - Give hope tempered with realism (honesty is an important element of these discussions, rather than being over optimistic. It maintains a patient's trust in her doctor which is important for the difficult treatment that lies ahead);

- The patient will need realistic reassurance about the future. Even when it is not possible to offer a cure, plans can be made for symptom control and support;
- Emphasize the importance of quality of life.
- Follow-up and closing up:
  - Summarize and check with patient;
  - Do not rush the patient to treatment;
  - Set up early further appointment, offer telephone calls;
  - Identify support systems; involve relatives and friends;
  - Offer to see daughter or others;
  - Make written materials available.

0   1   2   3   4

Appropriate conduct of consultation (sensitive, empathetic and reactive approach to the patient)   **[4]**

- Speak in a calm, quiet manner.
- Read the non-verbal clues; face/body language, silences, tears.
- Allow for 'shut down' (when patient turns off and stops listening) and then give time and space: allow possible denial.
- Keep pausing to give patient opportunity to ask questions; do not interrupt.
- Gauge patient's need for further information as you go and give more information as requested, i.e. listen to the patient's wishes as patients vary greatly in their needs.
- Encourage expression of feelings, give early permission for them to be expressed, i.e. *'How does that news leave you feeling'*, *'I'm sorry that was difficult for you'*, *'You seem upset by that'*.
- Respond to patient's feelings and predicament with acceptance, empathy and concern (use supportive non-verbal communication such as nodding and smiling, looks of concern, maintaining eye contact).
- Check patient's previous knowledge about information given.
- Elicit all the patient's concerns, e.g. *'Is there anything else worrying you?'*; *'Is there anything else you want to ask me?'*.
- Check understanding of information given, e.g. *'Is there anything you have not clearly understood?'*, *'Would you like to run through what you are going to tell your daughter?'*

0   1   2   3   4

Global score   **[4]**

0   1   2   3   4

Total: **/20**

Case notes

MRCOG II candidates are often fearful of the 'counselling' station – the angry or irrational patient/relative, the sad, distressed woman, etc. This is understandable as we all find dealing with these situations in our own professional, and for that matter, personal lives difficult. However, awareness of the following points will help you and give you confidence when approaching these difficult situations.

- **Giving space**. Even when bad news is expected, there will be an element of shock when the reality is put into words. This may last only a minute or two or a considerable time, depending on the seriousness of the news and its impact on the recipient. During this time, the patient is unlikely to retain any further information or even hear what is said to her. For this reason she needs space and time to think before any progress may be made. She may be still and silent and it is a temptation to fill this space with more information, reassurance and hope. What is required is that the silence is respected. If it goes on for a long time, you could say 'what you see': *'This news seems to be hard for you to take in', 'You seem to be quite shocked',* and *'I imagine you need some space to take it all in'*. These statements are all educated guesses, but are useful in that they break what may otherwise be a difficult silence, and also give the patient the opportunity to express her feelings, if she is ready.
- **Handling reactions**. Remember bad news will cause a shock reaction, even if it is expected. The patient will need time to absorb the news before she reacts to it. Ideally, the patient should be able to sit quietly, perhaps with a cup of tea, before disclosing her reactions, fears and worries. The shock may last only a few minutes, but sometimes longer – the patient's first reaction is an inability to talk about her feelings. Even in a busy clinic, some time should be allowed for bad news to be absorbed. Resist the temptation to fill the silence with more information, since it is unlikely that the patient will retain any more information at this time.
- **Listen attentively and acknowledge the patient's reactions**. Use open questions to encourage her to disclose her feelings, worries and concerns:
  - *'This must be difficult for you. Can you tell me how you are feeling?'*
  - *'I can see that you are angry, and I imagine I would be too in this situation.'*
  - *'You seem frightened. What is it that you find frightening?'*
  - *'Tell me more about how you are feeling just now.'*
  - *'What worries you most?'*
  - *'What does this news mean to you?'*

Remember to use non-verbal communication – facial expressions of concern, gestures, eye contact, etc. Comfort can be derived from simple supportive measures, such as appropriate touch, an empathetic approach or even a cup of tea, if this can be provided.

Further reading

The Breaking Bad News website (available at:
  www.breakingbadnews.co.uk).

Station 4 – Endoscopy/electrosurgery (Equipment, practical competencies)

Candidate's instructions

At this station you will have 14 minutes to answer questions and demonstrate practical competencies in relation to gynaecological surgery.

The examiner will ask you a series of questions about the practice of surgery and will provide you with relevant surgical instruments as part of the structured viva.

Marks will be awarded for:

- Your ability to answer the questions about surgical techniques;
- Your appreciation and understanding of safety issues;
- Your knowledge and application of surgical instrumentation;
- Your understanding and appropriate use of energy modalities.

Examiner's instructions

This is a structured viva and assessment of the candidate's practical skills. At this station, the candidate has 14 minutes to answer questions related to endoscopic surgery and to demonstrate the relevant competencies. You should ask the candidate the questions on your mark sheet and provide them with the endoscopes as appropriate. You can prompt the candidate if necessary, but this requirement should be reflected in the marks awarded.

You should have the following equipment:

- Hand-held surgical diathermy blade (A);
- 12° 8-mm cystoscope, obturator, outer sheath, biopsy forceps, Albarran bridge, short bridge (B);
- 30° single flow 5-mm continuous flow operative hysteroscope (C).

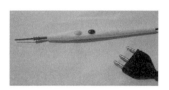
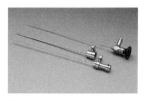
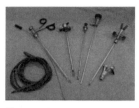

A   B   C

Questions to be asked:

Give the candidate the hand-held surgical diathermy blade:

1. Identify the instrument.
2. Describe how you would use it during abdominal entry and what diathermy settings/waveforms you would use.

Give the candidate the cystoscope and ancillary equipment
3. Identify the instrument, describe the key features and assemble it. What would you use it for?

Give the candidate the hysteroscope
4. Identify the instrument, describe the key features and assemble it. What would you use it for?
5. What are the advantages and disadvantages of using a 30° hysteroscope compared to a 0° instrument?
6. Describe what you would do if a poor view was obtained at hysteroscopy.

Structured mark sheet

Give the candidate the hand-held surgical diathermy blade.

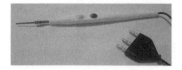

1. Identify the instrument. [1]
Hand-held surgical diathermy blade

0   1

2. Describe how you would use it during abdominal entry and what diathermy settings/waveforms you would use. [3]

- Incise skin – high power, pure cutting current.
- Incise subcutaneous tissue and rectus sheath and dissect rectus sheath off underlying rectus muscles (optimize performance by applying tension to the tissues) – pure cut, blended cutting current (1, 2, 3) or coagulation current.
- Haemostasis requires flat of the blade (increased surface area, reduce current density, less heat and coagulum formed and a blended current or coagulation waveform).
- Do not use it on the parietal peritoneum (risk of bowel injury).

0   1   2   3

Give the candidate the cystoscope and ancillary equipment.

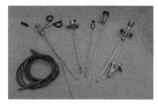

3. Identify the instrument, describe the key features and assemble it. What would you use it for? [3]

- 12° 8-mm rigid cystoscope, obturator, outer sheath, Albarran bridge, short bridge, biopsy forceps.
- Correct assembly.
- Diagnostic inpatient cystoscopy + directed bladder biopsies.

0   1   2   3

Give the candidate the hysteroscope.

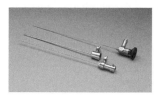

4. Identify the instrument, describe the key features and assemble it. What would you use it for? [3]

- 30° 5-mm continuous flow operative hysteroscope – identify inflow/outflow channels, 5 Fr operating channel.
- Correct assembly.
- Operative inpatient/outpatient hysteroscopy (polypectomy, myomectomy, sterilization (Essure™), IUCD retrieval, septoplasty).

0   1   2   3

5. What are the advantages and disadvantages of using a 30° hysteroscope compared to a 0° instrument? [2]

- **Advantages**:
  - Wider field of view so that rotation of the scope enlarges the field of view to the relevant areas;
  - Reduced torque on the cervix;
  - Aids operating (Versapoint™, use of mechanical ancillary instruments);
  - Enhances access to tubal ostia (aids sterilisation – Essure™).
- **Disadvantages**. More difficult to negotiate cervical canal for the inexperienced as the telescope will not be advancing in the direction that appears on the monitor [i.e. when it is aligned with the long axis of the endocervical canal, the dark circle representing it is located eccentrically at the bottom (6 o'clock position) or top (12 o'clock position) of the monitor].

0   1   2

6. Describe what you would do if a poor view was obtained at hysteroscopy. [4]

- Technical:
  - Check focus;
  - Check for debris/dirt on distal lens;
  - Check adequacy of light source (cable, light box, illumination settings).

- Inadequate distension:
  - Check tubing/connections/taps open/debris blocking the inflow/outflow channels;
  - Check inflow pressure – increase;
  - If patulous cervix or 'overdilated' cervix – close by application of vulsella to cervix.
- View obscured by bleeding/turbid fluid:
  - Improve irrigation (increase inflow pressure (> 70 mmHg intrauterine will allow transtubal flow and/or dilate the cervix to provide 'natural' outflow);
  - Consider changing to a larger diameter, continuous flow operating hysteroscope;
  - If using CO_2 change to fluid irrigation.

0   1   2   3   4

Global score [4]

0   1   2   3   4

Total: /20

Case notes

It is worth preparing for your exam by asking a scrub nurse to take you through a basic laparotomy instrument set and laparoscopy/hysteroscopy trays. You can spend 30 minutes familiarizing yourself with equipment, key features (e.g. vascular compression clamp vs an atraumatic tissue forcep), assembling endoscopes and examining their key features (laparoscopes, hysteroscopes, cystoscopes).

A formal resectoscope was not included in this question because, with the advent of second-generation endometrial semi-automated devices, their use is decreasing. However, if you have them in your department it would be worth spending a few minutes assembling them.

The next time you are performing a hysteroscopy or laparoscopy, think explicitly about what you are doing and how to rectify suboptimal surgical performance ('troubleshoot'). For example, this question could be about correcting a poor laparoscopic view (taps/connections/flow rates/insufflation pressures/light source, debris/dirt/focusing/blood absorbing light, smoke extractors/suction and irrigation for electrosurgery, etc).

An excellent short discourse on the principles of electrosurgery is available online (see Further reading) and will give those of you who are insecure about such questions more confidence for the forthcoming exam.

Further reading

Clark TJ, Gupta JK. 2005: Outpatient hysteroscopy: How to do it successfully. In: *Handbook of Outpatient Hysteroscopy: A Complete Guide to Diagnosis and Therapy*. London: Hodder Arnold.

Valleylab. Principles of Electrosurgery, 2005. (Available at: www.valleylab.com/education/poes/index.html).

Station 5 – Infertility (Case notes review)

Candidate's instructions

This is a preparatory station. Read the case notes, results and other documents provided. You may make notes on these sheets and take them with you to the next station where you will discuss the case with the examiner.

Marks will be awarded for:

Commenting on the notes, investigations, diagnosis and management steps, as well as answering the examiner's questions.

---

1. Referral letter

Rochdale Surgery
Mandela Road
Birmingham

22nd Feb 2005

Dear Doctor,

Would you please give an appointment to see Mr and Mrs Daly who have been trying to conceive for the past 7 years. Mrs Daly's periods are a little irregular. She has had a myomectomy under the care of Miss Patel at Ludwig General Hospital, but otherwise no significant history. Currently, she is on daily folate supplement. She is immune to rubella.

Thank you for your help.

Yours sincerely,

Dr Dodger

2. Outpatient notes

11/5/05	*New patient clinic*

11/5/05   *New patient clinic*
Couple seen together in clinic
Primary infertility for the couple for 7 years (secondary infertility for
Mrs Daly)

Mrs Daly
34 years; k = 4/30–45, irregular; periods light
Three miscarriages (all under 10 weeks, in 1994, 95 and 98 –
different partner)
? Had Lap and Dye (in Dubai) – ? 2003 – apparently one tube
blocked or swollen and scar tissue in the pelvis
Tried Clomid for 2 months (in Dubai) – ? Follicle tracking (had
several scans) – no pregnancy
PMH: myomectomy (for heavy periods)
LLETZ for CINII
Smokes 10/day
Alcohol – 16 units a week

Mr Daly
41 years
Fit and healthy
No prev pregnancies
Undescended testicles as a child – had surgery – Now OK; no
history of infection
No problems with erection/ejaculation
Non-smoker/no alcohol

O/E (*Mrs Daly*)
BMI 31
BP 120/70
Acne and hirsuitism (face and back)

Plan
Check FSH/LH
Check mid-luteal P
USS
SFA
See with results and arrange HSG

Dr Knight, SpR

22/6/05   FSH – 6
LH – 14
Oestradiol – 278

USS – see report
SFA – not done as Mr Daly could not produce (problem with getting the erection at the unit) – asked to try at home – but must bring specimen within 2 hours of production
PS: check TFTs and prolactin

Dr Loveless, SSHO

13/7/05   SFA – see report
Prolactin and TFTs – normal
Diagnosis and treatment options discussed – ICSI will be the best option
To check with GP re funding
D/W Mr Taylor (consultant) – offer ICSI

Dr Knight

3. LH, FSH and oestradiol lab report

Holyshire General Hospital NHS Trust
Mrs D Daly   DOB 17.04.1971   Patient number 1002569449
Lab report no: 223888
Date sample received 11.06.05

LH   14 U/L
FHS   6 U/L
Oestradiol   278 pmol/L

Date reported   15.06.05 Authorized by Dr Pathologist

4. Progesterone lab report

Holyshire General Hospital NHS Trust
Mrs D Daly   DOB 17.04.1971   Patient number 1002569449
Lab report no: 223993
Date sample received 23.05.05

Progesterone   18 IU (ovulatory range > 20 IU)

Date reported 28.05.05 Authorized by Dr Pathologist

5. Ultrasound report

Holyshire General Hospital NHS Trust
Mrs D Daly   DOB 17.04.1971   Patient number 1002569449
Date: 24/05/06
Ultrasound – pelvis
Indication: infertility

Report:
Uterus – 8 x 6 x 4 cm uterus; small (2 x 3 cm anterior wall fibroid – not distorting cavity)
ET = 5 mm; regular in outline
Right ovary – 23 x 18 x 14 mm (11 ml) – peripheral cysts – increased stroma
Left ovary – 24 x 15 x 14 mm (11 ms) – multiple peripheral cysts – increased stroma
No adnexa masses or free fluid

Scan and report by: MJC Cook

---

6. SFA report

Holyshire General Hospital NHS Trust
Mr C Daly   DOB 15.01.1964   Patient number 1002569582
Lab report no: 223993
Date sample received 28.06.05
Semen analysis

	Normal range
Volume = 3.6 ml	(≥ 2.0 ml)
Liquefaction time = 55 minutes	(within 60 minutes)
pH = 7.34	(≥ 7.2)
Sperm concentration = 4 million	(≥ 20 million/ml)
Motility (a+b) = 34%	[≥ 50% (grades a and b)]
Morphology = 4%	(15% or 30%)

Analysed and reported by Dr Davis

Station 6 – Infertility (Case notes review)

Marks will be awarded for:

Commenting on the notes, investigations, diagnosis and management steps, as well as answering the examiner's questions.

Examiner's instructions

The candidate has 14 minutes to discuss the given set of case notes. You should ask the candidate to discuss the case notes according to the marking scheme provided under the subheadings 'note-keeping', 'investigations', 'diagnoses' and 'management'.

Structured mark sheet

Comment on note-keeping [3]

- Clear entries; all entries dated and signed.
- Patient identification information missing from outpatient notes.
- Diagnosis not explicitly stated.
- Discussion about prognosis and treatment options (including risks/benefits) not documented.
- Information about care elsewhere *not* sought (e.g. details of myomectomy from Ludwig Hospital; details of laparoscopy from Dubai).

0   1   2   3

Comment on investigations [5]

Basic investigations are appropriate – appropriate to wait for SFA result and check for ovulation before arranging tubal patency test. However:
  - Tubal patency better checked with laparoscopy and dye test (RCOG recommendation; HSG or HyCoSy only if concurrent pathology not suspected – here there is suspicion of tubal disease including a hydrosalpinx, and adhesions);
  - When SFA abnormal, it should be repeated;
  - Was progesterone test timed correctly (irregular cycles)?
- Given the myomectomy, a cavity check (either with HyCoSy) or if undergoing a laparoscopy & dye, with a hysteroscopy, will be of value.

- Investigations for recurrent miscarriage are indicated (checking for APS, karyotyping, etc).
- If severe abnormality is confirmed on a repeat semen sample, consider checking the husband for karyotype and hormone profile.
- USS – should have also commented on the accessibility of the ovaries (for egg collection – especially with the history of adhesions).

0   1   2   3   4   5

Comment on diagnosis [3]

- Male factor and female factor.
- Female: probable tubal disease and anovulation (secondary to PCOS).
- Recurrent miscarriages.

0   1   2   3

Comment on management [5]

- ICSI is appropriate if the repeat SFA is also abnormal.
- Weight reduction (for Mrs Daly) would improve her chances with natural and assisted conception (NICE guidelines: BMI 19–29).
- Clomid induction (with or without IUI) is unlikely to be fruitful given the oligoasthenoteratozoospermia and tubal disease.
- If ICSI is what the couple are aiming for, then tubal assessment can normally be omitted (as ART bypasses the tube). However, laparoscopy to identify hydrosalpinx and salpingectomy if one found would improve success of ART.
- Mock embryo transfer may be required (as history of LLETZ).
- Mrs Daly to reduce alcohol intake (RCOG recommendation: No more than 1 or 2 units, no more than once or twice a week).
- If funding not available for ICSI, consider tubal surgery, ovulation induction (with Clomid, FSH, HMG, metformin or ovarian drilling), and IUI with prepared sperm (or donor sperm).
- As difficulty with sperm production, may consider sperm freezing as a back up to use on the day of egg collection.
- Complete documentation.
- Consents.

0   1   2   3   4   5

Global score [4]

0   1   2   3   4

Total: /20

Station 7 – Non-menstrual bleeding (history taking, communication, management)

Candidate's instructions

The patient you are about to see has been referred to your outpatient department by her GP.

Read the referral letter below and obtain a relevant history from the patient and discuss what examination and tests you feel are necessary with her. (The examiner will inform you of the examination findings on request.)

Dear Colleague

Re. Mary Jones

I would be grateful if you could see this 26-year-old teacher who is complaining of intermenstrual bleeding. She is very anxious and I would be grateful if you could see her and do the needful.

Yours sincerely

Dr G Halston MRCGP

Marks will be awarded for:

- Taking an appropriate history;
- Performing an appropriate examination and initial investigations and explaining the rationale for these interventions;
- Discussing likely diagnoses and appropriate management options.

Role player's instructions

You are Mary Jones, a 26-year-old teacher in a stable relationship. You have been on the combined oral contraceptive pill (Microgynon) for 3 years and remember to take this as prescribed. You have no medical problems of note, but smoke 15 cigarettes a day. You are nulliparous and have no immediate fertility plans, but have had a first trimester surgical termination of pregnancy in the past.

Your menstrual cycles are regular and not heavy, but you have noticed light intermittent intermenstrual bleeding (spotting) over the last 6 months, which occurs at any time during the pill cycle. You have also noted some light bleeding after sexual intercourse on occasions recently. Although you have no pelvic pain or dyspareunia, you have noticed a heavy, clear, non-odorous vaginal discharge.

You have never had a smear.

You are very worried about your symptoms, especially because your mother died 2 years ago from endometrial cancer.

Examination findings – prominent cervical ectopy, friable but no cervical lesions. Otherwise normal lower genital tract and pelvis.

Examiner's instructions

Candidates have 14 minutes to demonstrate the following:

- Ability to take an appropriate history.
- Ability to perform an appropriate examination and initial investigations, and explain the rationale for these interventions.
- Ability to discuss likely diagnoses and appropriate management options.

Structured mark sheet

History [6]

- Nature of IMB – duration, pattern, timing, amount and frequency of bleeding, and normal 'cycle' withdrawal bleeds.
- COC and compliant.
- Elicit PMB history and ascertain its nature – amount, intermittent, not associated with dyspareunia.
- Vaginal discharge.
- Smear history and smoking.
- Elicit TOP and family history.

0   1   2   3   4   5   6

Examination and investigations [3]

- Abdominal and pelvic examination:
  - Inspection of the vulva/vagina (candida);
  - Inspection of cervix (ectopy, polyps, suspicious lesions, friability).
- Cervical smear.
- Genital tract swabs (to include HVS, endocervical and chlamydial).
- (Consider pelvic ultrasound).

0   1   2   3

Diagnosis and management [7]

- IMB – breakthrough bleeding on COC but need to await swab results to exclude genital tract infection (*Chlamydia trachomatis*, candida).
- PCB – may be related to cervical ectopy, but need to obtain smear result to exclude dyskaryosis and swabs to exclude genital tract infection.
- Vaginal discharge – cervical ectopy, genital tract infection.
- Endometrial polyp.
- Reassure if tests all normal. Explain that cervical ectopy (exposed columnar cells) is physiological but can be more pronounced with the COC.
- Try changing COC to one with a different progestogen; consider Cerazette POP.
- Consider treatment of cervical ectopy (cauterization, cryotherapy, LLETZ) only as a second line and explain evidence for efficacy limited.
- Treat genital tract infection appropriately with antibiotics, antifungals, and arrange contact tracing via GU clinic if STI.
- Repeat smear ± colposcopy if abnormal smear. Outpatient hysteroscopy + uterine polypectomy if polyp on scan.

0   1   2   3   4   5   6   7

Global score [4]

0   1   2   3   4

Total: /20

Case notes

Non-menstrual bleeding is common. Over a 6-month period, 7–10% of women will experience IMB and 2–4% PCB. Although the vast majority of women with unscheduled, non-menstrual bleeding do not have any significant underlying pathology, such symptoms tend to provoke a disproportionate amount of anxiety in patients and their doctors.

Routine referral is indicated for recurrent and persistent symptoms in association with a normal pelvic examination. Urgent referral should be considered where IMB/PCB symptoms are found in association with pelvic pain or dyspareunia or an abnormal pelvic examination (suspect appearance or lesions on vulva, vagina and cervix, friable cervix/contact bleeding, pelvic mass not thought to be fibroids) or abnormal cervical smear (squamous or glandular dyskaryosis, BNA, HPV, mild atypia on repeated testing).

There are many potential causes of IMB. However, in this case 'physiological bleeding' [e.g. mid-cycle – peri-ovulatory hormonal fluctuations (occurs in 1–2% of normal cycles; luteal phase defect – inadequate progestogenic endometrial support) is not relevant because she is on the COC and there is no cyclical pattern to IMB. Serious endometrial disease (cancer and hyperplasia) is unlikely in a woman under 40 years with regular cycles on the COC. Trauma and vulvo-vaginal pathology (urogenital atrophy, dermatoses, etc) are unlikely causes of PCB in view of her age and absence of dyspareunia.

The main potential diagnoses are thus:

1. Breakthrough bleeding in association with the COC, which is common initially even in women with good compliance and no drug interactions/GIT disorders;
2. Genital tract infection – friable cervix may suggest cervicitis, past history of TOP and discharge (although malodorous and clear suggests physiological);
3. Cervical dyskaryosis should be considered as a cause of PCB as she is over 25 years of age, has not had a cervical smear and is a smoker (note: up to 17% of women with PCB will have CIN).

Uterine polyps can cause endometrial dysregulation and lead to IMB/PCB, but this diagnosis is unlikely in women under 40 years with regular cycles. An ultrasound scan is relatively non-invasive and may be useful here to provide additional reassurance in view of her mother's history of uterine cancer. A hysteroscopy ± endometrial biopsy is not indicated in view of the low prevalence of endometrial pathology, unless the scan reveals an abnormal endometrium.

Management will involve review of investigations and reassurance if all normal. As symptoms are not self-limiting (> 6 months), it is reasonable to change the COC preparation to one with a different progestogen to see if it gives better endometrial support, absorption, etc. Although POPs are less effective than the COC and are associated with DUB, Cerazette POP prevents ovulation in 95% of women and so may provide better cycle control and the lack of exogenous oestrogen may reduce the size of the cervical ectopy.

Prominent cervical ectopies may be excised or ablated using a variety of outpatient methods and CIN treated by LLETZ. It should be noted, however, that although a modest association between presence of cervical ectopy and vaginal discharge has been shown, no such association has been found with PCB or IMB. Thus such intervention, especially in young, nulliparous women, should be considered second line for refractory cases.

Further reading

Clark TJ, Gupta JK. 2005: Intermenstrual and postcoital bleeding, abnormal cervical smears and vulvo-vaginal disorders. In: *Handbook of Outpatient Hysteroscopy: A Complete Guide to Diagnosis and Therapy*. London: Hodder Arnold: Chapter 11.

Connolly A, Jones SE. 2004: Nonmenstrual bleeding in women under 40 years of age. *TOG* **6**:153–158 (available at publications.thedriveris.com: 2052/RCOG/doi/pdf/10.1576/toag.6.3.153.26997).

Station 8 – Diabetes and pregnancy (Communication, counselling, management)

Candidate's instructions

You are about to see Shobna Agarawal, a 29-year-old solicitor, who has attended the outpatient department for pre-pregnancy counselling. She was diagnosed with Type 2 diabetes mellitus last year, which is being controlled on the oral hypoglycaemic glibenclamide.

Your task is to conduct relevant comprehensive pre-pregnancy counselling and address any concerns or misunderstandings the patient may have. You have 14 minutes.

Marks will be awarded for:

- Demonstration of good communication skills;
- Clear and comprehensive discussion of the implications of diabetes and pregnancy;
- Appropriate advice regarding management of pregnancy;
- Addressing the patient's concerns.

Role player's instructions

You are Shobna Agarawal, a 29-year-old married solicitor. You have never been pregnant before.

You were diagnosed with Type 2 diabetes mellitus last year and this is being controlled with diet and oral medication. You are generally fit and well, with no other medical or surgical history. You take vitamin supplements daily.

You have been having the contraceptive injection (Depo-Provera) for the last 3 years for fertility control. Your periods are infrequent and very light. You last had a cervical smear 7 years ago.

You have a family history of high blood pressure (your mother and father are both on treatment for this). You drink alcohol and smoke socially.

You are keen to start a family, but are very worried about this because you have heard that many babies born to diabetic mothers are abnormal. You have also heard that it is better to deliver the baby by a planned elective caesarean section.

Examiner's instructions

This is a structured viva. Listen to the consultation and award marks according to your mark sheet for how well this is conducted and for the clarity of discussion. Pay particular attention to the candidate's ability to:

● Demonstrate good communication skills.
● Discuss the implications of diabetes and pregnancy.
● Give appropriate advice regarding subsequent management of pregnancy.
● Address the patient's concerns.

You can prompt the candidate if necessary, but this requirement should be reflected in the global marks awarded.

Structured mark sheet

Pre-pregnancy counselling [6]

● **Context – risks of diabetes in pregnancy:**
  – Diabetes mellitus (Types 1 and 2) is the most common pre-existing medical condition to affect pregnant women with a frequency of 2–5/1000 pregnancies;
  – Pregnancy can affect diabetes and vice versa.

TABLE 12.3 Risks to mother and fetus of diabetes in pregnancy

Risks to mother	Risks to fetus
Miscarriage	Congenital abnormality/miscarriage
Hypoglycaemia/hyperglycaemia	Macrosomia
Premature labour	Growth restriction
Retinopathy	Birth trauma (shoulder dystocia)
Hypertension/pre eclampsia	Neonatal hypoglycaemia
Nephropathy	Neonatal polycythaemia
Caesarean section	Neonatal hypocalcaemia

- **Context – importance of diabetic control pre-conceptually and antenatally:**
  Pre-conceptual care does improve outcome (and is cost-effective). Specifically:
  - Optimal metabolic control reduces the risk of miscarriage, congenital malformations [especially NTDs; congenital anomaly rates background 1–2.5%; diabetes 4–10% (OR 2.0–4.0)];
  - Optimal metabolic control reduces the risk of an unhealthy baby;
  - Give an outline of routine management during pregnancy: attendance at joint diabetic clinics with a named obstetrician and physician and standardized protocols for management; tight blood sugar control (glycaemic targets) – diet and insulin, self-management requirements, hospital assessments; advice re hypoglycaemia management to patient and partner; close surveillance of fetal growth and wellbeing, blood pressure, urine (infection, proteinuria, glycosuria and ketones).

0   1   2   3   4   5   6

Pre-pregnancy obstetric advice – general [8]

- Folic acid 5 mg/day (at least 3 months pre-conception and until 12 weeks' gestation).
- Stop smoking.
- Reduce/cease alcohol intake.
- Review all medications (including complementary) for safety in pregnancy – avoid vitamin A (teratogenic).
- Check BP.
- Check rubella (? and varicella) immune status.
- Cervical smear (not performed within last 3 years).
- FBC (? anaemia), blood group and antibodies.

Pre-pregnancy obstetric advice – specific

- Contraception:
  - Stop DMPA – as oligo-menorrhoeic and used DMPA for 3 years, it may take up to 1 year for fertility to return;
  - Use barrier contraception (or POP/COC) for the next 3 months to allow for folate supplementation and establishment of tight diabetic control.
- Diabetic control and pre-pregnancy glycosylated haemoglobin level (HbA1c) – pregnancy should be delayed until HbA1c < 8.0% (assessment of chronic hyperglycaemia – associated with increased risk of miscarriage).
- Oral hypoglycaemic agents are contraindicated during pregnancy + may not allow adequate control. Glibenclamide will need to be stopped and

conversion under the care of a diabetic physician to insulin prior to conception.
- Tight blood sugar control – targets:

HbA1C	< 6–7%
Preprandial plasma glucose (fasting)	< 5 mmol/L
Postprandial (2 hour) plasma glucose	< 6.7–7.8 mmol/L

One way of achieving this is with the basal-bolus regimen – one long- or intermediate-acting insulin at night to provide basal control and bolus doses before meals.
- Dietary advice – dietician/nurse specialist.
- Self-management – control blood sugars, self-injection, finger prick blood glucose monitoring (mornings, after meals).
- Aware of dangers of:
  - Hypoglycaemia management must be reviewed, including glucagon use by the partner. Early morning hypoglycaemia more common in early pregnancy – suggestions for dealing with morning sickness could be discussed;
  - Hyperglycaemia and ketoacidosis.

Pre-pregnancy obstetric advice – diabetic complications screening

- Nephropathy:
  - U&Es, Cr (Cr > 150 μmol/L – poorer pregnancy outcome);
  - Urine for proteinuria estimation and creatinine clearance (< 50 ml – poorer pregnancy outcome).
- Retinopathy:
  - Refer to ophthalmologist for an eye examination conducted through dilated pupils;
  - Proliferative retinopathy predictive of fetal outcome and risk of progression (10% if absent; 50% if present);
  - Retinopathy requiring treatment should be dealt with prior to pregnancy (laser photocoagulation).
- Consider the possibility of macrovascular disease (e.g. IHD, CVA) and formally investigate if a possibility.

Pre-pregnancy obstetric advice – conception
Early review when pregnancy is confirmed.

0   1   2   3   4   5   6   7   8

Concern regarding mode of delivery – general [2]

- C/S can be safer in certain circumstances, namely when the baby is very big (macrosmia) and there is a risk of difficulty delivering the shoulders (shoulder dystocia) or if there is significant fetal compromise (IUGR).
- However, vaginal delivery is safe and to be encouraged (as in women without diabetes) to avoid the unnecessary risks of surgery.

Concern regarding mode of delivery – gestation at delivery

- NICE recommends that women who have pregnancies complicated by diabetes should be offered induction of labour prior to their estimated date for delivery (40 weeks). This is because of increased potential problems in the late third trimester:
  - A higher perinatal mortality rate (OR 3–5), which incorporates an increased rate of late fetal death (stillbirth rate five times that of the general population);
  - Increased rate of other complications necessitating preterm delivery (e.g. pre-eclampsia);
  - Increased potential for birth trauma associated with increased fetal size. Infants of diabetic mothers are particularly prone to brachial plexus injury caused by shoulder dystocia (IOL of term pregnancies in women with diabetes is associated with a reduced risk of macrosomia and does not appear to increase the risk of caesarean section or neonatal morbidity, cases of which are rare and mild).
- In general women with optimal glycaemic control and no complicating factors (microvascular disease, hypertension, fetal macrosomia, IUGR, poor glycaemic control, smokers) do not generally require delivery before 40 weeks, with the method depending on obstetric factors. If an elective caesarean section is to be performed, it should be at 39 weeks.
- Patients with one of the complicating factors mentioned above should be delivered at 38–39 weeks, or earlier if indicated. Elective caesarean section should be performed at 38 weeks.

Concern regarding mode of delivery – mode of delivery

- In the absence of complications, a vaginal delivery should be planned for 38–40 weeks. The caesarean section rate is usually 2–3 times the background rate at 40–60%.
- If EFW at the time of delivery is < 4000 g, vaginal delivery is usually appropriate unless there are other obstetric indications for caesarean section.
- If EFW at the time of delivery is > 4250 g, elective caesarean section should be strongly considered because of the risk of shoulder dystocia.

- If EFW at the time of delivery is 4000–4250 g, the decision about the route of delivery should be discussed with the patient, taking into account the risks for the particular patient.

0   1   2

Global score   [4]

0   1   2   3   4

Total: /20

Case notes

Diabetes and pregnancy is a fertile ground for clinical questions/scenarios as examiners can explore a number of issues in relation to communication and knowledge of management (pre-pregnancy, screening, antenatal care, delivery, post-partum, neonatal).

Diabetes types:

- Type 1 – this results from autoimmune destruction of the insulin-producing islet cells. The condition therefore requires insulin and tends to present in childhood.
- Type 2 – this results from a state of relative insulin resistance. It was formerly referred to as 'maturity onset' but this is no longer the case, especially in obese women and those of Indo-Asian background.

Do not forget the potential for macrovascular (coronary arteries, the aorta) as well as microvascular complications (neuropathy, nephropathy, retinopathy:

St Vincent Declaration Goals and Targets aim to achieve a pregnancy outcome for women with diabetes that equates with that of women without diabetes. Unfortunately the outcomes of stillbirth, congenital abnormalities, neonatal death rate and perinatal mortality remain higher than in the background population, although the results have improved. Tight diabetic control and pre-pregnancy counselling is integral to this goal. It is estimated that only 30% of women with known diabetes attend for pre-pregnancy care.

Further reading

Knox E, Dunne F. 2001: Perinatal Review – Diabetes in Pregnancy. The Perinatal Institute. (Available at: www.perinatal.nhs.uk/reviews/diabetes/diabetes_intro.htm).

Station 9 – Dyspareunia and vulval disorders (History taking, communication, management, viva)

Candidate's instructions

The patient you are about to see has been referred to your outpatient department by her GP.

Read the referral letter below and obtain a relevant history from the patient. The examiner will then ask you a series of related questions.

Dear Colleague

Re. Mary Stevens

I would be grateful if you could see this 28-year-old pharmacist who is complaining of dyspareunia since getting married last year. She is keen to start a family and this complaint is preventing her from doing this and is putting a strain on her relationship. I would be very grateful for your opinion and advice on further management.

Yours sincerely

Dr A Prasad DCH DRCOG MRCGP

Marks will be awarded for:

- Taking an appropriate history;
- Ability to answer the examiner's questions.

Role player's instructions

You are Mary Stevens, a 28-year-old pharmacist.

You were a virgin when you got married 12 months ago. Sexual intercourse has been a problem ever since your sexual 'debut'. Specifically you find penetration very uncomfortable and experience severe burning pain in the vagina during sex such that only rarely are you able to continue. You find now that you are tense prior to sex and this is compounding the situation and affecting your ability to be aroused. You do not enjoy sex as a result and have never had an orgasm. You do not have pain in your abdomen, the pain you experience is very much 'superficial', i.e. vaginal and on the 'outside'.

You have a good relationship with your loving partner, but he is becoming increasingly distant and avoiding intercourse with you because 'he doesn't want to hurt you'. You are upset and worried that he will leave you because of your inability to satisfy him or to start trying for a family.

In addition to the painful sex, you have noticed recently that you are experiencing itching and soreness around the outside of the vagina, especially premenstrually. You get 'thrush' and urinary tract infections occasionally.

Your periods are fine. You have never tried using tampons but use sanitary towels for menstrual hygiene.

You have no medical problems that you are aware of, in particular no history of skin diseases. The only surgical history you have is that you did have a 'Bartholin's cyst' drained from the lower vagina as a student 7 years ago. You do not smoke or drink alcohol.

Examiner's instructions

Familiarize yourself with the candidate's and role player's instructions. Allow the candidate 7 minutes to take the relevant history and then ask the questions on your mark sheet. You may prompt the candidate, but this should be reflected in the marks you give.

You should have: a photograph depicting a vulva with lichen sclerosus.

Questions you should ask:

1. You examine the patient. On initial inspection the vulva/vagina appears normal. What differential diagnoses are you considering at present and what further examination findings may suggest these diagnoses?
2. Your examination and investigations (lower genital tract swabs) are negative. Briefly outline potential management strategies?
3. This is a picture taken from a 66-year-old woman with vulval symptoms of burning itching and superficial dyspareunia with postcoital bleeding. Describe the features seen. What diagnoses would you consider and how would you confirm or refute this?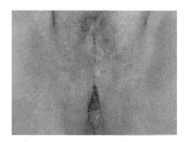
4. The biopsy reveals lichen sclerosus. How would you treat this?

Structured mark sheet

Relevant history   [8]

● Define dyspareunia and/or concomitant sexual dysfunctions:

- Where is the pain located?
- When is the onset of the pain? (before, entry, vaginal, deep or after).
- Is it pruritic, burning or aching in quality?
- What is the chronological history? If multiple pain sites, which came first?
- Is it situational or positional?
- Has it been lifelong or acquired?
- Are there other sexual dysfunctions such as arousal, lubrication or orgasmic difficulties?
- What treatments have been attempted?
- Explore potential gynaecological causes:
  - Are there vaginal symptoms, including discharge, burning or itching?
  - Does patient have a history of STDs, especially HSV?
  - Is there an obstetric delivery history of lacerations, episiotomies or other trauma?
  - Is there an abdominal or genitourinary (incontinence) surgical or radiation history?
  - Has the patient had prior gynaecological diagnoses, including endometriosis, fibroids or chronic pelvic pain?
  - What is the patient's current contraception method and is there any history of intrauterine device use?
- Explore potential medical causes:
  - Is there evidence or history of chronic disease, collagen vascular disorders, autoimmune diseases – diabetes mellitus, thyroid?
  - What are the patient's medications: alternative, prescribed, over-the-counter?
  - Is there alcohol or drug use?
  - Does the patient experience bowel or bladder symptoms?
  - Is there evidence of skin disorders such as eczema, psoriasis or other dermatitis?
- Obtain psychosocial information:
  - What is the patient's view of the problem?
  - Has the problem been present in other relationships?
  - Are the partners able to discuss the problem? If so, what actions have they tried?
  - (Is there any history of sexual or physical abuse?) May be inappropriate at first visit or perhaps introduce if examination findings suggestive, e.g. vaginismus.
  - To what extent are other life stressors a factor?
  - Is there evidence of depression or anxiety disorders?
  - What would be considered a satisfactory treatment outcome?

0   1   2   3   4   5   6   7   8

1. **You examine the patient. On initial inspection the vulva/vagina appears normal. What differential diagnoses are you considering at present and what further examination findings may suggest these diagnoses?** [2]

Superficial dyspareunia in the absence of vulvar skin disorders:
- Essential dyspareunia – none (diagnosis of exclusion);
- Vulvodynia [dysesthetic (essential) vulvodynia] – (NAD or mild erythema, marked tenderness);
- Vulvar vestibulitis (subset of vulvodynia) (erythema, intensity varies; margins distinct or vague; exquisite tenderness on touch of cotton-tipped applicator);
- Vaginismus (palpable spasm of vaginal musculature; difficulty inserting speculum);
- [Atrophic tissue or impaired lubrication (visual inspection of pubic hair, labial fullness, integrity of vaginal mucosa, vaginal depth; vaginal mucosal friability, fissures – atrophy unlikely in woman of this age without symptoms of premature ovarian failure)];
- Infection – (acute/chronic infections – candida, BV, TV, HSV) – (discharge, typical lesions, in lower genital tract, tenderness over urethra/anterior vaginal wall if urethritis);
- Vulvovaginal cysts/varicose;
- Bartholin gland – recurrence, inflammation, scarring from previous surgery (tender/erytherma ± lesion over Bartholin gland openings).

0   1   2

2. **Your examination and investigations (lower genital tract swabs) are negative. Briefly outline potential management strategies?** [2]

- Reassurance (no STI, normal anatomy, other young women have this condition, etc)
- General measures:
  - Avoid scratching ('itch–scratch cycle');
  - Avoid soap, shampoo and bubble bath;
  - Use aqueous cream or emulsifying ointment as a soap substitute;
  - Avoid tight fitting garments;
  - Use cotton underwear and avoid synthetic materials;
  - Avoid use of spermicidal cream/impregnated condoms;
  - Use bland, non-irritating moisturizer such as aqueous cream/petroleum jelly;
  - After urinating or having a bowel movement, clean the genital area gently with absorbent cotton or antiseptic wipes. Wipe from front to back (vagina to anus);

– Tampons rather than sanitary towels;
– Avoid overexertion, heat and excessive sweating;
– Lose weight if appropriate.
- Specific measures:
  – KY jelly, water based products (e.g. Replens), baby oil during intercourse (topical oestrogen cream in older women with atrophic vaginitis);
  – Topical local anaesthetic prior to intercourse;
  – Trial of topical steroids – break 'itch–scratch cycle';
  – Change in diet (avoid allergenic agents – caffeine beverages, tomatoes, peanuts, dairy);
  – Psychosexual counselling (psychological evaluation, CBT, exploration of negative sexual attitudes, sexual ignorance – discussion of foreplay, arousal phase mechanics, expected sensations, use of mechanical dilators/vibrators).

0   1   2

3. This is a picture taken from a 66-year-old woman with vulval symptoms of burning itching and superficial dyspareunia with postcoital bleeding. Describe the features seen. What diagnoses would you consider and how would you confirm or refute this? **[2]**

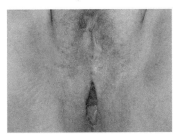

- LSA – leukoplakia – an abnormal condition characterized by white spots or patches on mucous membranes. The typical lesion appears as white, atrophic, 'parchment paper-like' or crinkled paper patches of the vulvar skin, occasionally accompanied by marked contracture with narrowing of the introitus (hence the old term kraurosis vulvae). Note the white epithelium with atrophic labia majora and narrowing of the vestibule.
- Consider:
  – Non-neoplastic disorders of the vulva (squamous cell hyperplasia);
  – Vulval dermatoses;
  – VIN;
  – Vulval cancer.
- Confirm – vulvoscopy + biopsy.

0   1   2

4. The biopsy reveals lichen sclerosus. How would you treat this?   [2]

- Scabicide crotamiton (Eurax) cream.
- Topical steroid suitable for long-term use [graduated topical steroids – maintenance (allow absorption)]
- Follow-up (malignant potential).
- Surgery (caution because of high recurrence rate 50% – WLE/simple vulvectomy)
- Other – 2% topical testosterone, oral retinoids, 5-FU.

0   1   2

Global score   [4]

0   1   2   3   4

Total: **/20**

Case notes

We are all uncomfortable with taking a sexual history and generally we do it inadequately. The sensitive and embarrassing nature makes it a difficult task and the general gynaecological outpatient clinic is not the appropriate environment to explore the issues in detail. As a gynaecologist you can identify and treat vulvovaginal 'organic' disorders underlying superficial dyspareunia, but psychological factors, especially in the presence of vaginismus, are frequently at play (such as childhood sexual abuse), so referral for psychosexual counselling is important when it is felt this is indicated.

Vulvodynia – classically the patient reports numerous unsuccessful visits to various doctors for relief of ongoing vulvar burning or rawness. In such a case, vulvodynia should be considered. The cause of vulvodynia is unknown, but some of the many theories suggest chronic irritation from vulvovaginal candidiasis, vestibular papillomatosis caused by human papillomavirus, and reactions to chemicals used to treat condylomata. Among the clinically defined subsets of vulvodynia are vulvar vestibulitis and dysesthetic (essential) vulvodynia. In vulvar vestibulitis, the patient complains of entrance dyspareunia, and the vulvar vestibule appears erythematous. The sensation of burning or stinging is elicited with the touch of a cotton swab. In dyesthetic vulvodynia, there are no abnormal clinical findings. Although the mechanism of pain is uncertain, studies have shown a strong association between psychological distress and dyesthetic vulvodynia. One theory is that stress, through neurological pathways, heightens sensitivity of nerve fibres.

In questions about 'deep dyspareunia', again a sensitive approach would be required, providing reassurance where necessary. The differential diagnoses to consider would be endometriosis and pelvic adhesions, adnexal pathology, retroverted uterus, chronic cervicitis, pelvic congestion, pelvic relaxation – prolapse, urethral disorders, cystitis, interstitial cystitis, IBS.

Think about the investigations and treatment you would offer:

- Long-term follow-up of patients with lichen sclerosus is required because a small proportion will develop vulval cancer.
- Bartholin's cyst – due to obstruction of the duct draining the Bartholin gland leading to retention of secretion and resultant cystic dilatation of the duct. The condition presents as a palpable mass in the lower third of the vestibule, posterolateral to the introitus. It occurs at all ages and may cause local discomfort and dyspareunia.
- Many conditions involving the vulva – benign, premalignant and malignant – present as white patches. It is very crucial for patient management to distinguish between these lesions. Biopsy is therefore very important and indicated for the diagnosis of all white lesions of the vulva.
- Squamous cell hyperplasia – presents as thick grey–white plaques of the vulva and occurs in women between 30 and 60 years old. Areas lacking a keratin layer appear red. The patches may be circumscribed or diffuse. Any part of the vulva, adjacent thighs, perineum or perianal skin may be involved. The lesions are pruritic and scratching adds trauma and chronic inflammation. Histologically there is epithelial thickening with acanthosis and hyperkeratosis. Parakeratosis may occur on the surface. The lesion is not premalignant, but if dysplasia is present, it can be associated with a low risk for development of squamous cell carcinoma.
- The treatment of vulval cancer and VIN is unlikely to be a clinical OSCE question, but could arise in the written exam. That said, you should be aware of the symptoms/signs suggestive of the condition and the differential diagnoses.

Further reading

RCOG. 2006: *Management of Vulval Cancer*. London: RCOG Press (Available at: www.rcog.org.uk/resources/Public/pdf/vulval_cancer.pdf).

RCOG. 2003: *Lower Genital Tract Neoplasia – Study Group Recommendations*. London: RCOG Press. (Available at: www.rcog.org.uk/index.asp?PageID=308).

Station 10 – Neonatology (Viva, practical competencies – emergencies)

Candidate's instructions

At this station you will have 14 minutes to answer questions about the care of the newborn baby.

You perform a ventouse-assisted delivery of a healthy term baby for failure to progress. As you are delivering the baby, the student midwife who is present and who takes the baby informs you that the baby appears 'a bit flat' and is not crying. How would you manage this situation?

This is a structured viva. The examiner will ask you a series of questions about relevant neonatology.

Marks will be awarded for:

Your ability to answer questions about the obstetric care of the newborn baby.

Examiner's instructions

At this station, the candidate will have 14 minutes to discuss the obstetric management of the newborn baby. You should ask the candidate the questions in the order they appear on your mark sheet.

Questions to be asked:

1. What is your immediate management?
2. The baby is fine and responds quickly to simple resuscitative measures. You notice a bruised caput succedaneum over the occiput. You visit mum and baby on the postnatal wards later that day and notice the baby is jaundiced. What are the likely causes?
3. What tests would you expect to have been done to investigate early pathological jaundice?
4. The baby's jaundice settles down within the next 2 days without treatment other than rehydration. On day 4 the baby is noted to be 'jittery' and not feeding well. Neonatal seizures are diagnosed by the paediatrician. What are the most likely causes?
5. Mum also complains of lethargy, headache, nausea and feeling feverish. Her temperature is 38° C. On systemic enquiry she reports a heavy, offensive lochial loss and also a painful and tender right breast. On examination the breast appears red, indurated and tender and pelvic examination reveals a tender, bulky uterus with a closed external cervical os. What diagnoses do you suspect and how would you investigate and treat this situation?

Structured mark sheet

1. What is your immediate management?   [6]

- Call for help – student midwife to call senior midwife/call paediatrician.
- **Assessment:**
  - Respiration – the newly born infant should establish regular respirations in order to maintain HR > 100 bpm;
  - Heart rate – determined from direct palpation of cord, apex beat or with stethoscope. Peripheral pulses are often difficult to feel. If no pulsation is felt on palpation of the cord, do not assume there is no heart beat but auscultate the chest. The HR should be > 100 bpm in a well newly born infant;
  - Colour – the well newly born infant should be able to maintain a central pink colour in room air.
- **Management:**
  - Environment – prevent heat loss by drying infant, warm towels, place on resuscitaire, availability of equipment (O_2 supply, suction, bag and mask circuit, laryngoscope, ET tubes);
  - Stimulation – most infants respond to stimulation with movement of extremities. Appropriate stimulation includes drying the face or flicking the bottom of the feet. If meconium is present in a non-vigorous infant, suction under direct vision. Delay tactile stimulation to avoid gasping in the infant with an oropharynx full of particulate meconium;
  - Airway – the head should be in a neutral or slightly extended 'sniffing' position. Suction should not exceed –100 mmHg. It should be limited in depth to 5 cm below the lips to clear inhaled vernix, blood or meconium;
  - Breathing – attend to adequate inflation and ventilation before oxygenation. The rate for assisted ventilation is 60 bpm. Tidal volume is assessed clinically, i.e. adequate chest excursion with each breath. Few infants require immediate intubation. The majority of infants can be managed with bag and mask ventilation;
  - Circulation – in the majority of infants establishment of adequate ventilation will restore circulation. Begin chest compressions either for absent HR or HR < 60 for 30 seconds;
  - Aim for approximately a ratio of 90 chest compressions to 30 breaths/ minute (3:1; 120 events/minute) – count 'one-and-two-and-three-and-breathe'. (The 'two-thumb' technique is preferred. Both thumbs meet over the sternum with fingers around the chest wall. The sternum should be compressed to one-third of the antero-posterior chest dimension);
  - Advanced management should be undertaken by a paediatrician unless

adequately trained [intubation, medications via umbilical venous catheter or ET (adrenaline/naloxone), lines, fluids, etc];
- Attend to mother (once help has arrived and according to wellbeing of the mother).

0   1   2   3   4   5   6

2. The baby is fine and responds quickly to simple resuscitative measures. You notice a bruised caput succedaneum over the occiput. You visit mum and baby on the postnatal wards later that day and notice the baby is jaundiced. What are the likely causes? **[2]**

- Haemolysis – with excessive production of bilirubin exacerbated by bruising from ventouse:
  - Common causes of haemolysis – ABO incompatibility, Rh immunization, sepsis (decreasing order of probability);
  - Rarer causes of haemolysis – other blood group incompatibilities, red cell enzyme defects, e.g. G6PD deficiency, red cell membrane defects, e.g. hereditary spherocytosis.
- Hepatitis (rare).
- Note: 'Physiological' jaundice is the most common cause of jaundice after 24 hours (begins day 2–5) and usually resolves within 10 days; more pronounced with breastfeeding. Jaundice after this time – consider breast milk jaundice, continued poor milk intake, haemolysis, infection (especially UTI), hypothyroidism (all unconjugated hyperbilirubinaemia) or hepatitis (infection – TORCH, syphilis; metabolic disorders, galactosaemia)/biliary atresia (conjugated hyperbilirubinaemia).

0   1   2

3. What tests would you expect to have been done to investigate early pathological jaundice? **[2]**

- Total and conjugated serum bilirubin concentration (SBR).
- Maternal blood group and antibody titres (if Rh negative).
- Baby's blood group, direct antiglobulin (Coombs') test (detects antibodies on the baby's red cells), and elution test to detect anti-A or anti-B antibodies on baby's red cells (more sensitive than the direct Coombs' test).
- Full blood examination, looking for evidence of haemolysis, unusually-shaped red cells, or evidence of infection.

0   1   2

4. The baby's jaundice settles down within the next 2 days without treatment other than rehydration. On day 4 the baby is noted to be 'jittery' and not feeding well. Neonatal seizures are diagnosed by the paediatrician. What are the most likely causes? **[2]**

The most common identifiable disorders are:

- Hypoxic–ischaemic encephalopathy (49%);
- Cerebral infarction (12%);
- Cerebral trauma (7%);
- Infections (5%);
- Metabolic abnormalities including hypoglycaemia (3%);
- Narcotic drug withdrawal (4%).

0   1   2

5. Mum also complains of lethargy, headache, nausea and feeling feverish. Her temperature is 38° C. On systemic enquiry she reports a heavy, offensive lochial loss and also a painful and tender right breast. On examination the breast appears red, indurated and tender, and pelvic examination reveals a tender, bulky uterus with a closed external cervical os. What diagnoses do you suspect and how would you investigate and treat this situation? **[4]**

- Endometritis and mastitis.
- Investigation and treatment – general. As mum unwell and temperature >38° C, then perform FBC, CRP, blood cultures and commence broad-spectrum antibiotics to include aerobic and anaerobic cover.
- Investigation and treatment – mastitis:
  - Breast milk culture, ± ultrasound (diagnose abscess if suspected clinically or symptoms/temp persist – refer to breast surgeon for either percutaneous aspiration or open drainage);
  - Early management – maintain breastfeeding, effective milk removal, analgesia: paracetamol or NSAID;
  - Later management – if symptoms are not resolving within 12–24 hours, antibiotic treatment may be required [penicillinase-resistant penicillins, e.g. flucloxacillin (cephalexin if allergic) used for bacterial infections caused by *Staphylococcus aureus*; safe, does not accumulate in breast milk and levels in breast milk are undetectable 6 hours after dosage].
- Investigation and treatment – endometritis:
  - LGT swabs (role of endocervical cultures is controversial); MSU helps exclude UTI;

- TVS (if not responding to initial treatment or placenta 'ragged' at delivery – exclude RPOC);
- Broad-spectrum antibiotics as aetiology is polymicrobial; a mixture of aerobic and anaerobic organisms is usually found (e.g. Cef and Met, Augmentin)

0   1   2   3   4

Global score   [4]

0   1   2   3   4

Total: /20

Case notes

Neonatology is specificd on the MRCOG II syllabus. It is unlikely you will be tested in detail on this during the OSCE, but common problems such as illustrated in this example may be addressed. Some of you may have done some neonatology as an SHO. For those who have not, a quick review of neonatal care from a basic undergraduate textbook or an overview tutorial from a paediatric colleague should suffice.

Further reading

NHS Quality Improvement Scotland. Routine Examination of the Newborn Best Practice Statement, 2004. (Available at: www.nhshealthquality.org/nhsqis/files/20219%20BPS_Newborn%20.pdf).

Station 11 – Infection and the fetus (chicken pox) (Communication, management)

Candidate's instructions

You are in your antenatal clinic and Jim Bradshaw, a local GP, phones you to ask for advice regarding a pregnant woman who has brought her 6-year-old son to the surgery with a rash that has been diagnosed as chicken pox. The woman is currently 38 weeks' pregnant and is extremely anxious because she is unsure whether she has ever had chicken pox herself. She is also concerned because she and her son met a pregnant friend the day before whilst walking in the park.

Describe the advice you would give to the GP regarding management of this situation.

Marks will be awarded for:

- Obtaining relevant additional information from the GP;
- Giving clear advice about further management;
- Explaining the implications of chicken pox infection in this situation.

Examiner's instructions

Candidates have 14 minutes to demonstrate the following:

- Ability to obtain relevant additional information.
- Ability to give clear advice about further management.
- Ability to explain the implications of chicken pox infection in this situation.

Structured mark sheet

Additional information [2]

- Mother – Is she at risk of severe disease, e.g. chronic lung disease, heavy smoker, immunosuppressed (on steroids, HIV)?
- Contact with pregnant friend – How long were she and her son in contact and what did this entail?

0   1   2

Advice and further management [9]

- Advise patient to check with her mother regarding any childhood history of chicken pox and assume immunity with a definite history. Reassure.
- If uncertain or negative past history then send urgent serology to check for IgG antibody to varicella zoster (may be able to use serum stored from antenatal booking) and if negative give varicella zoster immunoglobulin (VZIG). Consider use of prophylactic aciclovir.
- The patient should be advised to notify her GP early if a rash develops and subsequently report promptly any symptoms suggestive of maternal complications (e.g. respiratory or neurological symptoms, haemorrhagic rash, bleeding) or new skin lesions after 6 days.
- Contact with friend – reassure that infection risk minimal in outdoor environment and > 90% chance that friend is immune. Only potential risk is if friend is non-immune and prolonged face-to-face contact. Friend should then attend her GP for advice, serology and VZIG if appropriate.
- Avoid contact with other pregnant women and neonates for the next 3 weeks.

0   1   2   3   4   5   6   7   8   9

Implications of infection [5]

- Reassure the GP/mother – in most women chicken pox infection causes no lasting harm to them or their babies.
- Mother – serious respiratory (pneumonia), neurological (encephalitis) or haemorrhagic complications can occur, but these are rare in healthy women.
- Fetus – serious fetal infection (fetal varicella syndrome) is extremely rare after 28 weeks of pregnancy
- Newborn – the newborn acquires protective maternal antibodies if born > 7 days after maternal rash so unlikely to develop severe infection. Infection of the newborn is common where the maternal rash develops between 7 days before and 7 days after birth. Serious infection of the newborn is rare, especially if at-risk babies are identified and appropriately treated (VZIG, aciclovir).

0   1   2   3   4   5

Global score

0   1   2   3   4

Total: /20

Case notes

Chicken pox is caused by the varicella zoster virus. 90% of women > 20 years old are immune (i.e. have protective antivaricella serum antibodies). The virus is highly transmissible by respiratory droplets or close contact with an infected person. Exposure to the virus and onset of characteristic rash is 10–21 days (incubation period). The affected person is infectious from 48 hours before the onset of the rash until crusting of the lesions.

The risks associated with exposure to chicken pox are:

- **To pregnant woman**: Severe infection – chicken pox pneumonia, which can be fatal (respiratory symptoms, e.g. SOB, cyanosis, haemoptysis), encephalitis causing cerebellar ataxia and haemorrhagic complications. Risks higher in immunocompromised, chronic lung diseases, heavy smokers and those in the latter half of pregnancy.
- **To fetus**: There is no evidence of an increased incidence of spontaneous miscarriage or intrauterine death. Risk of fetal varicella syndrome (segmental skin loss and scarring, reduced birth weight, limb hypoplasia, paresis, microcephaly, neurological anomalies and ophthalmic lesions) is negligible after 28 weeks' gestation.
- **To neonate**: Mother with chicken pox transmits virus to her infant around the time of delivery in circumstances where the infant lacks the protection of maternal antibodies. The development and transfer of maternal antibodies takes 7 days from the time of the rash. Thus the baby is at significant risk (60%) of developing varicella infection if the maternal rash develops between *7 days prior and 7 days after* delivery.

Significant exposure comprises face-to-face conversation for 5 minutes, over 15 minutes in the same room or living in the same household. VZIG is recommended in pregnant women who have: significant exposure in the infectious period [48 hours prior to onset of rash until vesicles crust over (usually by day 5–7)] in the *last 10 days*; no past history of chicken pox; and antibody negative. Oral aciclovir is not licensed in pregnancy and is generally not recommended for prophylaxis. Only consider its use in women with significant risk factors (e.g. immunosuppressed, smokers, early VZIG not received, second half of pregnancy). Varicella vaccine is a live attenuated virus and is therefore contraindicated in pregnancy.

Pregnant woman with chicken pox:

- Should avoid contact with other pregnant women and neonates, and be counselled on the risk of fetal varicella syndrome (negligible after 28 weeks' gestation).

- Can take paracetamol to relieve fever, headache or myalgia, but *not* NSAIDs (premature closure of the ductus arteriosus > 30 weeks).
- Can take antihistamines after the first trimester (e.g. chlorphenamine) but *not* during breastfeeding.
- Oral aciclovir can be used to treat/attenuate symptoms but there is no evidence for effectiveness if the mother presents after 24 hours of the first observed lesion. Intravenous aciclovir should be given in a specialist isolation facility if severe disease develops. VZIG has no place in treatment once chicken pox has developed.
- Generally there is no need for hospital admission unless symptoms suggest complications or new skin lesions after 6 days. However, hospital assessment should be considered where there are risk factors (smoker, lung disease, immunosuppressed, latter half of pregnancy). Women close to term should be considered for hospitalization because of the risks of haemorrhagic complications or varicella infection of the newborn. Discuss with local neonatologist and virologist.
- Where relevant and practical, delivery should be delayed until 5 days after the onset of maternal illness to allow for passive transfer of antibodies that could protect the baby from infection.

Further reading

Chickenpox, pregnancy and the newborn. 2005: *Drug Ther Bull* **43**:6972.
RCOG Green Top Guideline. Chickenpox in pregnancy (13), June 2001. (Available at: www.rcog.org.uk/resources/Public/pdf/Chickenpox_No13.pdf).

Station 12 – Medical disorders/complications of pregnancy (Viva, management)

Candidate's instructions

At this station you will have 14 minutes to answer questions about medical disorders and complications in pregnancy.

This is a structured viva. The examiner will ask you a series of questions about medical problems that may arise during pregnancy.

Marks will be awarded for:

Ability to answer questions about medical disorders and complications that may arise during pregnancy.

Examiner's instructions

At this station, the candidate will have 14 minutes to discuss questions about medical disorders and complications that may arise in pregnancy. You should ask the candidate the questions in the order they appear on your mark sheet.

Questions to be asked:

1. A woman presents to the early pregnancy assessment unit at 10 weeks' gestation complaining of nausea and vomiting. What clinical findings would make you want to admit her to hospital?
2. What investigations would you perform and why?
3. You decide that she has severe hyperemesis gravidarum with dehydration, ketosis and deranged LFTs. How would you manage this woman?
4. She has a persistent tachycardia despite adequate fluid rehydration. She has a raised free T4 and free T3 and suppressed TSH. What are the likely diagnoses?
5. How would you manage this woman antenatally and what pregnancy-related complications would you look out for?
6. At 31 weeks' gestation this woman is referred by her community midwife with itching associated with mildly elevated liver transaminases and bile acids. You examine her and find her to be normotensive with evidence of scratching on her palms and feet, but no rash or proteinuria. What diagnosis do you suspect and how would you confirm this?

Structured mark sheet

1. A woman presents to the early pregnancy assessment unit at 10 weeks' gestation complaining of nausea and vomiting. What clinical findings would make you want to admit her to hospital? **[2]**

- History – nausea and vomiting non-responsive to simple measures, such as reassurance and dietary changes (small, frequent, light meals with high-carbohydrate or high-protein content – avoid offensive odours, fatty foods, spicy foods, iron supplements).
- Examination – tachycardia, postural changes in BP and pulse, decreased skin turgor, weight loss of at least 5%.
- (Investigations) – electrolyte imbalance, ketosis (> 1+ ketones).

0   1   2

2. What investigations would you perform and why? **[2]**

- Urine for ketones; MSU to exclude UTI.
- FBC, U&Es, LFTs, RBG, as a one-off screen.
- USS to exclude trophoblastic disease or multiple pregnancy.
- TSH if suggestion of hyperthyroidism (heat intolerance, tachycardia, palpitations, palmar erythema, emotional lability and goitre).

0   1   2

3. You decide that she has severe hyperemesis gravidarum with dehydration, ketosis and deranged LFTs. How would you manage this woman? **[4]**

- IV fluids (dextrose solutions may stop fat breakdown) and electrolyte restoration (monitor U&Es, LFTs).
- Nutritional supplements – pyridoxine (vitamin B_6), thiamine (vitamin B_1).
- Antiemetics (parenteral).
- Steroids.
- Antacids, H_2 antagonists.
- Consider referral to hepatology.
- (Enteral feeding – for patients who fail to respond to the above management).
- Continue treatment until patient can tolerate oral fluids and until test results show few or no ketones in the urine.

0   1   2   3   4

4. **She has a persistent tachycardia despite adequate fluid rehydration. She has a raised free T4 and free T3 and suppressed TSH. What are the likely diagnoses?** [1]

Hyperemesis gravidarum and thyrotoxicosis (Graves disease, 95%).

0   1

5. **How would you manage this woman antenatally and what pregnancy-related complications would you look out for?** [4]

- **Management**:
  - Examine for goitre, repeat TFTs and thereafter monthly TFTs as newly diagnosed thyrotoxicosis;
  - Refer to endocrinologist for assessment and treatment [carbimazole (aplasia cutis), PTU – preferable, aim for lowest dose to achieve clinical euthyroid with free T4 at upper end of normal], ? beta-blockers for symptoms – tachycardia, sweating, tremor;
  - Serial scans for growth/fetal wellbeing (IUGR) ± fetal neck imaging (for goitre – only poorly controlled newly diagnosed thyrotoxicosis) ± FBS (fetal TFTs!).
- **Complications**:
  - Mother – usually nil if well controlled; if poorly controlled – thyroid crisis ('storm' – hyperthermia, mental disorientation, atrial fibrillation, cardiac decompensation) and heart failure, particularly at the time of delivery; rare – retrosternal extension of goitre – tracheal obstruction (dysphagia, stridor, problems with intubation);
  - Baby – miscarriage, IUGR, prematurity, perinatal mortality, fetal/neonatal thyrotoxicosis.

0   1   2   3   4

6. **At 31 weeks' gestation this woman is referred by her community midwife with itching associated with mildly elevated liver transaminases and bile acids. You examine her and find her to be normotensive with evidence of scratching on her palms and feet, but no rash or proteinuria. What diagnosis do you suspect and how would you confirm this?** [3]

- **Diagnosis** – obstetric cholestasis of pregnancy.
- **Confirmation** – exclude other causes of abnormal LFTs:
  - Viral screen for hepatitis A, B, C, EBV, CMV;
  - A liver autoimmune screen (smooth muscle and antimitochondrial antibodies) for chronic active hepatitis and primary biliary cirrhosis;
  - Liver ultrasound.

0   1   2   3

Global score [4]

0   1   2   3   4

Total: /20

Case notes

Hyperemesis gravidarum is characterized by persistent, severe nausea and vomiting that begins before 20 weeks' gestation, resulting in dehydration, electrolyte imbalance, ketosis and weight loss of at least 5% of the pre-pregnant weight. Hyperemesis affects about 1% of pregnancies compared to the more common occurrence of milder nausea and vomiting ('morning sickness'), which can occur in 50-70% of pregnancies.

The epidemiological study suggesting a causative role for obstetric cholestasis in stillbirth is methodologically flawed, so without further research the significance of OCP will remain hotly debated. The recent RCOG guidance clearly states that routine intensive fetal surveillance has not been shown to improve outcome and neither has maternal interventions, such as the use of UDCA. However, the presence of abnormal LFTs in pregnancy warrants investigation to exclude incidental (PBC, hepatitis) or pregnancy-related liver disease (OCP, AFLP, PET) testing.

Thyrotoxicosis is associated with a 48% fetal mortality if left untreated in pregnancy. hCG has some thyroid stimulating activity and can cause biochemical hyperthyroidism with normal or low TSH levels. So, if there are no clinical features of thyrotoxicosis (weight loss, exophthalmos, tachycardia, restlessness), then no treatment is necessary.

Further reading

Edelman A, Logan JR. Pregnancy, hyperemesis gravidarum. E-Medicine, 2004 (Available at: www.emedicinc.com/EMERG/topic479.htm).

Nelson-Piercy C. 2001: Thyroid and parathyroid disease. In: *Handbook of Obstetric Medicine*. Oxford: Taylor & Francis, Chapter 6.

RCOG Green Top Guidelines. Obstetric Cholestasis (43), Jan 2006. (Available at: www.rcog.org.uk/index.asp?PageID=1348).

Index